The Uses of Reminiscence:
New Ways of Working
with Older Adults

The *Journal of Gerontological Social Work* series:

The Uses of Reminiscence: New Ways of Working with Older Adults

Marc Kaminsky
Editor

The Haworth Press
New York

The Uses of Reminiscence: New Ways of Working with Older Adults has also been published as *Journal of Gerontological Social Work*, Volume 7, Numbers 1/2, March 1984.

The Haworth Press, Inc., 28 East 22 Street, New York, NY 10010

Library of Congress Cataloging in Publication Data
Main entry under title:

The Uses of reminiscence.

    "Has also been published as Journal of gerontological social work, volume 7, numbers 1/2, March 1984"—T.p. verso.
    "A bibliography of reminiscence and life review [by] Harry R. Moody": p.
    Includes bibliographical references.
    1. Gerontology—Biographical methods. 2. Aged, Writings of the, American. 3. Social work with the aged—United States. I. Kaminsky, Marc, 1943-
II. Journal of gerontological social work.
HQ1061.U76   1984   305.2'6'0922   84-4520
ISBN 0-86656-272-9
ISBN 0-86656-285-0 (soft)

For Dr. Robert Butler
who gave us the idea

and for Nancy Larson Shapiro
who helped put it into practice

The Uses of Reminiscence: New Ways of Working with Older Adults

Journal of Gerontological Social Work
Volume 7, Numbers 1/2

CONTENTS

II. CONCEPTS AND PRACTICES

III. APPENDIX

IV. NOTES

SHELDON TOBIN, PhD, *Director, Ringel Institute of Gerontology, Albany, NY*
TERESA JORDAN TUZIL, MSW, *Consultant on Aging, New York, NY*
EDNA WASSER, MSW, *Consultant, Fellow, Gerontological Society, Miami, FL*
MARY WYLIE, PhD, *Professor, Department of Social Work, University of Wisconsin, Madison, WI*

Contributors

BARBARA BARACKS is the author of three books, *Poems Out of Place, Notes #1-23*, and *No Sleep*. Her fiction and poetry have been included in several anthologies. Her art criticism, book reviews, and journalism have appeared in *The Village Voice, Artforum, The Soho News, Ms., The Feminist Review*, and other publications. She has taught writing and video workshops to elementary school children and older adults.

JANET BLOOM is associate editor of *Architectural Forum* and *Architectural Record*. Her poems and essays have appeared in *The American Poetry Review, The New York Quarterly, Parnassus, Arts*, and other magazines. She has taught writing in elementary schools and senior centers. Ms. Bloom holds an MFA from Goddard.

ROSE DOBROF is Professor of Social Work at the Hunter College School of Social Work and director of the Brookdale Center on Aging. She edited *Social Work Consultation in Long-Term Care Facilities* and co-authored *The Maintenance of the Family Relationships of Old People in Institutions: Theory and Practice*. Her papers on aging have been widely published. She is a Fellow of the Gerontological Society, and Editor-in-chief of the *Journal of Gerontological Social Work*. She holds a DSW from the Columbia University School of Social Work.

GEORGE GETZEL is Associate Professor and chairman of the group work sequence at the Hunter College School of Social Work. His articles on group work and aging have been widely published in professional journals. He is currently editing two books on geriatric social work practice, and is the practice editor of the *Journal of Gerontological Social Work*.

ROLAND LEGIARDI-LAURA is the founding director of the Poets Overland Expeditionary Troop (POET), a traveling performance group and small press distribution outlet. Two anthologies of his students' writing have been published by Teachers & Writers Collaborative, and his own fiction and poetry have appeared in *Out There, Ah Noi, Sunbury, Words to Go Anthology*, and other publications.

MARC KAMINSKY is the founding director of the Artists & Elders Project and co-director of the Institute on Humanities, Arts and Aging at the Brookdale Center on Aging of Hunter College. His poems and essays have appeared in *The American Scholar*, *Midstream*, *The New York Times*, The *Journal of Gerontological Social Work*, and many other publications, and his work has appeared in several anthologies, including *The New Old: Toward a Decent Aging* and *Voices within the Ark: the Modern Jewish Poets*. His four books of poems include *A Table with People* and *Daily Bread*. He is also the author of *What's Inside You It Shines Out of You*, a book about conducting poetry workshops with old people.

SUSAN MILLER LONDON teaches gerontology at Touro College. She is the founding director of the Theatre for Older People at the Joseph Jefferson Theatre Company, and has taught older adults at a number of colleges, including the New School for Social Research Creative Arts Center for Older Adults. Ms. Miller holds master's degrees in theatre and psychology, and is a doctoral student at Columbia University Teachers College.

HARRY R. MOODY, JR. is the director of academic affairs at the Brookdale Center on Aging and co-director of the center's Institute on Humanities, Arts, and Aging. In addition, he directs the National Council on Aging Center on Education, Leisure, and Continuing Opportunities for Older People. He has published widely on the life cycle and philosophies of education for older adults, as well as on late-life styles of aging artists. He holds a PhD in philosophy from Columbia University, and teaches courses in philosophy at Hunter College and New York University School of Continuing Education.

SUSAN PERLSTEIN has taught theatre, dance, and movement at senior centers and colleges in the New York area, and has considerable professional experience in the theatre and modern dance. She founded the Mass Transit Street Theatre, and is currently director of the Hodson Senior Drama Group, which was the subject of a documentary film on the use of oral history in creating plays.

ROCHELLE RATNER is the author of seven books of poetry. The most recent is *Combing the Waves*; she is co-editor of *Hand Book*, a literary magazine; managing editor of the *American Book Review*. Ms. Ratner has taught poetry workshops to older adults in senior centers and hospitals.

LUCILLE WOLFE began her social work career in 1930 when she joined the staff of the Jewish Social Service Agency. She earned her MSW at the Pennsylvania School of Social Work and, after years of working with refugees, became involved in marriage and family counseling at the Jewish Family Service and the Community Service Society. She currently leads a writing and reminiscing workshop for older adults at a church on Manhattan's Upper West Side.

DALE WORSLEY conducted workshops with retired seamen at the National Maritime Union and edited the resulting oral history, *Lives at Sea: Stories of Retired Seamen*. He is the author of a novel, *The Focus Change of August Previco*, and is currently working on a series of radio plays with the theatre company Mabou Mines.

GRACE WORTH is a field representative for the Humanities Program of the National Council on the Aging. She has taught college courses in writing, children's literature, gerontology, and child care and development. Ms. Worth spent four years organizing rural families in Fayatteville, Ohio, helping them create and run their own family and child care center. She holds a master's degree in English and an ABD (All But Dissertation) in American Literature from Notre Dame.

JEFFREY CYPHERS WRIGHT is the editor of *Compass*, a magazine which publishes writing by older adults, and of Hard Press, which publishes poetry postcards. He edited *Over the Years*, an anthology of poems and stories by older people in his workshop at the Countee Cullen Library in Harlem. Mr. Wright is a member of the Poets Overland Expeditionary Troop, and the author of *Employment of the Apes*. His work has appeared in *Voices*, *Contact II*, and *Teachers & Writers Magazine*.

BILL ZAVATSKY has taught writing for the Teachers & Writers Collaborative since 1971. Between 1977 and 1979, he taught writing at the University of Texas at Austin. His book reviews, articles, and criticism have appeared in the *New York Times Book Review*, *Rolling Stone*, the *American Book Review*, and many other magazines. He co-edited *The Whole World Catalog II*, an arts education sourcebook, and is the author of *Theories of Rain and Other Poems*.

Acknowledgments

This book grew out of the work of the Artists & Elders Project, a workshop program for older adults which I organized under the auspices of Teachers & Writers Collaborative. For me, the meaning of the project as a whole became associated with eight particular voices—contradictory, laughing, immediate, hurt, hooked, mournful, inquiring, raw, needling, apologetic, plunging towards insight, overwhelmed, rainy, tactful, indignant, rippling with assurance, haunted, concerned: voices of the people in the Astoria Workshop. None of us came away from this experience unchanged. For three years, I spent nearly every Tuesday morning with Frances Arluck, Josephine Dreher, Margaret Friedman, Aurelia Goldin, Israel Raphael, Irene Salamon, Julia Schubert, and Lillian Steinberg. To say I'm grateful to them for sharing their reminiscences, their writings, and their lives with me doesn't fully convey my feeling or the tone of the group: it was an immense pleasure to participate in that passionate exchange.

There is a second group of people with whom I worked closely: the directors of Teachers & Writers Collaborative. The project would not have happened without Steve Schrader's vision, Neil Baldwin's hard work, and Nancy Larson Shapiro's special blend of generosity and wisdom. Their dedication enriched the lives of both elders and artists: this book is dedicated to them.

The group of artists—Barbara Baracks, Janet Bloom, Neil Hackman, Roland Legiardi-Laura, Susan Perlstein, Dale Worsley, and Jeff Wright—included two "artists at social work": Lucille Wolfe, a veteran of fifty years in the field, and Carolyn Zablotny, who directed a senior center on the Upper West Side of Manhattan. All of them approached the project with a spirit of adventure, intent on making a voyage of discovery. They went out to libraries, union halls, senior centers, nursing homes, and casework agencies, where they organized and conducted the workshops they describe in these pages. Vigilant, resourceful, persistent, they were quick to discern the hidden currents in their new situations; and, by letting themselves be guided by what was already in the wind, they became effective guides, enabling older people to speak of what William

Carlos Williams called "the strange phosphorus of life, nameless under an old misappelation." In their hands, the inarticulate mess of rush and routine and fragments of spirit mixed up with husks of dead language yielded shapes of meaning.

While planning and editing this book, I consulted with each of them. Barbara Baracks and Janet Bloom made valuable suggestions on two of my pieces. I showed various parts of the manuscript to other colleagues at Teachers & Writers Collaborative and the Brookdale Center on Aging. I'm grateful for the comments and criticisms I received from Miguel Ortiz, Jill Crabtree, Alan Feldman, Mark Weiss, Sue Willis, Madelaine Santner, Dina McClellan, Rochelle Ratner, Rick Moody, and Rose Dobrof. The Brookdale Center on Aging supported work on this book by providing release time for Joanne Scavella, who typed part of the manuscript, and for Karen Schwartz, who assisted with the copyediting. The preparation of the book was also supported by grants from the Literature Program of the National Endowment for the Arts.

The primary sources of support—both for the book and for the Artists & Elders Project—came from the New York Foundation and the Vincent Astor Foundation. I'm deeply grateful to Madeline Lee of the New York Foundation, and to Brooke Astor and Linda Gillies of the Vincent Astor Foundation, for their caring and knowledgeable involvement in every phase of the project. The project's parent organization, Teachers & Writers, was funded in part by the New York State Council on the Arts and the National Endowment for the Arts.

A number of the essays which were written for this book first appeared in Teachers & Writers. These include: "The Passion of Recollection," by Barbara Baracks; "Snug Harbor: Workshops at the National Maritime Union," by Dale Worsley; "Tapping the Legacy," by Jeff Wright; "Heal, Body, Heal: Invocations to Health and Hope," by Rochelle Ratner; "Minerva's Doll," by Janet Bloom; "Realities of Aging: Starting Points for Imaginative Work with the Elderly," by Susan Miller London; and "A Kind of Odyssey," by Lucille Wolfe. "Poetry, Groups, and Old People," by George Getzel, was first published in the Journal of Gerontological Social Work.

M.K.

Introduction:
A Time for Reclaiming the Past

Within recent years the publication of Alex Haley's *Roots* and the television series based on the book were dramatic events—widely read, watched, analyzed. The book and the series were interesting, in and of themselves. But they were also representative of a dramatic upsurge of interest in autobiography, in sociological and anthropological studies of ethnic roots, in "Life review" and reminiscence in the service of the ego integrity of older people, in the use of informal remembrances of ordinary people as tools of social historians.

One can only speculate about why these last decades of the twentieth century should be a time for reclaiming the past. Some see young people's interest in their own family history as an effort to find continuity and stability in an age of change and anomie. Others call attention to the politics of ethnicity: if ethnic background is one consideration in the division of the social pie of resources, then one's own ethnicity becomes important in one's claim to a piece of the pie. Technology is also an influence. I read an essay by a musicologist who wrote about how he felt as a young man when works of the masters recorded by the great musicians of our century were first produced. Before then, he wrote, the sounds of a performance were lost—except in memory—when the performances ended. With technology the performance endures as inspiration and enjoyment for millions of people now and for future generations.

Perhaps tape recorders and word-processing machines are to the spoken word what the phonograph is to music: they make it possible for us to preserve the voices of our mothers and fathers telling us the history of their times. Technology expands the possibilities, and interest rises with the dawning recognition of the possibilities. In the field of aging, interest began with the publication in 1963 of a seminal paper by Dr. Robert Butler, founding director of the National Institute on Aging.[1] It is not often that one paper has so immediate and profound an effect. I was then a very junior social worker on the staff of a home for the aged. I remember well being

xvii

taught by our consulting psychiatrists and the senior social work staff about the tendency of our residents to talk about childhood in the shtetls of East Europe or arrival at Ellis Island or early years on the Lower East Side of New York. At best, this tendency was seen as an understandable, although not entirely healthy preoccupation with happier times, understandable because these old and infirm people walked daily in the shadow of death. At worst, "living in the past" was viewed as pathology—regression to the dependency of the child, denial of the passage of time and the reality of the present, or evidence of organic impairment of the intellect.

It was even said that "remembrances of things past" could cause or deepen depression among our residents, and God forgive us, we were to divert the old from their reminiscing through activities like bingo and arts and crafts.

And then the Butler paper came out and was read and talked about and our world changed. The Life review became not only a normal activity; it was also seen as a therapeutic tool. In those years we had also discovered Eric Erikson, who wrote of the developmental tasks of old age, of the struggle to escape despair and achieve ego-integrity, of the necessity to accept "the historical inevitability" of one's life. What was, was, and alternative paths were no longer possible.

We put the *aperçu* of Erikson together with Butler's more systematic and clinically tested formulations: the Life review was the ground on which the old waged the struggle for integrity; it was here that they reexamined and came to terms with the Was. In a profound sense, Butler's writings liberated both the old and the nurses, doctors and social workers; the old were free to remember, to regret, to look reflectively at the past and try to understand it. And we were free to listen and to treat rememberers and remembrances with the respect they deserved, instead of trivializing them by diversion to a bingo game.

We learned in these encounters with the old and their memories that we were always talking about both personal and public events. One old man spent his days unspeaking and almost motionless. He had left his village in Poland to come to New York as a young man, promising to send for his wife and baby daughter as soon as he could get a job and save up the money for the passage. That day never came, and his wife and by then grown-up daughter were among the six million Jews killed in the Holocaust. Now in 1963 he sat, an old man alone in a home for the aged, crushed by the burden of his unspeakable guilt.

How could anyone understand his pain and try to find an anodyne for it if his story remained private, isolated from the history of the pogroms of the late 1800s and the immigrants' experiences, including their failures, in the New World? We tried: he was not the only man who had broken his promises to those he left behind, whose dreams had been killed in the sweatshops of the garment industry and who, safe and alive, in a home for the aged in the Bronx in 1963, was nonetheless a victim of the Holocaust.

We tried, but it remained for Marc Kaminsky to bring together the public and private, the story and the history in a vibrant, seamless whole. In this book he presents his own writings and those of an extraordinary collection of people, whom, by dint of the passion of his conviction and the elegance of his work, he has recruited to the cause—writers, teachers, philosophers, social workers, artists and older people themselves. They tell their stories: they talk about how poets and artists and social workers and historians and old people can together recount the past and live in a present made true in the recounting.

Rose Dobrof

The Uses of Reminiscence: New Ways of Working with Older Adults

I. MODES OF PRACTICE

Transfiguring Life:
Images of Continuity
Hidden Among the Fragments

Marc Kaminsky

1. RECAPTURING HIDDEN FIGURES OF THOUGHT

"A year from now," I said, as I handed around the blue looseleaf notebooks, "I will collect these again, but they'll be filled—with the events of your daily life, sudden encounters with the past, unbidden memories, dreams, angry letters, quatrains, quotations that are part of the world the writer salvages in his notebook, dialogues with God, or with yourselves, grammar exercises, sessions with the dead who continue to speak to you, stories about times of danger, milestones in your life, places of refuge, invocations to the wind, whatever you like . . . Whatever grabs you, puzzles you, aches to get said—let it come into this book. You can always remove it: that's what makes a looseleaf notebook a license to say whatever you like. At the end of our first year together, when I collect these journals, there's a good chance you'll have discovered what you have to say as a writer, as well as your distinct way of saying it."

There were seven women and a man in the writing workshop at the JASA Astoria Senior Center. During the course of the "journal project," each one—with an empty book to fill—began to approach the world as a writer: predatory, receptive, curious, curatorial, they sought to find in their everyday lives the raw materials for stories and poems. Because of the keener attention they paid to them, their lives grew richer.

When the year was up, and I was reading through their journals, I made a startling discovery. I had sat through two life reviews without being quite aware of what I was hearing. Week after week, Margaret Friedman and Irene Salamon read their journal entries aloud in the workshop. I felt in their narratives a suggestiveness, an aura, which distinguished them from other—flatter—retellings of the past. But only in my study, when I reexamined these particular sequences of reminiscences, did I understand their hidden relation to each other and to the life of each writer.

From the journals of Margaret Friedman and Irene Salamon I learned that, although the *concept* of the life review is readily grasped, the life review itself usually eludes us, like shapeshifting Proteus, the Old Man of the Sea who rolls from change to change and thereby slips through the hands of those who try to capture him. By allowing the older people in the workshop to discover their own subjects, in their own forms, I enabled them to reveal what neither they nor I knew when we started out: that the life review doesn't take any form we might have expected. Fragmentary, half-submerged, moving quickly from one disguise to another, the hidden figures of thought whose presence I dimly sensed in the workshop now appeared clearly before me. I was face to face, at last, with living examples of the process that Robert Butler had postulated more than twenty years ago. Here was the heightened awareness of death, and the elegiac feeling-tone; here was the return of repressed memories, associated with conflict and guilt, now recaptured with tremendous sensory vividness; here, finally, was that transfiguring of experience which, like Emily Dickinson's "certain slant of light," leaves "internal difference/Where the meanings are."

We had been fortunate: two of the people in the workshop happened to be undergoing life reviews during the year of our "journal project." And fortunate that we'd been granted enough time for something as slow and intermittent as a profound process of change to run its course. Fortunate, too, that both Margaret Friedman and Irene Salamon were sufficiently open to their experience to allow the life review process to govern their writing. If we had not been favored by these circumstances, we could not have discovered, through our collaboration, how one of the most significant events in late life manifests itself. It is something we almost always miss.

2. THE BIRTHDAY GIFT

Here are five entries from the journal of Margaret Friedman:

February 26, 1979—Piano

Remember the ads, "They all laughed when I sat down to the piano"? As a child, I took piano lessons. I practiced because my mother naturally reminded me of my responsibility.

I always had one eye on the clock. I would much rather read than play the piano. I've always loved music; while I could recognize someone else's flat notes, I never heard mine.

This morning, it must have been the early part, I dreamed I had been playing the piano beautifully—no errors, timing, everything perfect. I woke up, remembering all the details but I smiled to myself. I go to the piano these days only to dust it.

April 4, 1979—An Old Song

The radio is softly playing "April Showers," an old song from my childhood. As I sit having my breakfast, I am transported to the apartment we lived in on East 80th Street in Yorkville.

As clearly as if it were now, I can see the round golden oak table with the high-back chairs, the buffet, Mama's sewing machine by the window, and the player piano; this was our dining room. We had music rolls which were put on a roller which we pumped with our feet and lo and behold! we could listen to opera, the classics, dance to the popular tunes of the day.

My mother and sister would sing and Papa would whistle. They all had pretty good voices but I never felt mine was much good, so I enjoyed listening to them. Those were happy days. What a song can do for your memory!

Fridays, when Mama would be up very early in the morning to prepare the dough for her Friday baking, the dish with the dough was covered with a feather pillow to keep it warm so that it would rise; no steam heat in the apartment in those days, only the warmth and the delicious aroma when my sister and I came home for lunch. As soon as we reached the first floor, we could smell the cake. By mid-afternoon all the neighbors had fresh cake. The machine near the window was covered with plates of goodies as was the buffet. When we came home at three o'clock you could choose coffee cake with chocolate or what we call Danish today with cheese, nuts, apricots, or prune jelly. Nothing but nothing that I eat today tastes half as good as what Mama gave us on Friday afternoon with our milk.

Funny what one song can do to your mind.

April 20, 1979—Springtime and Lilac Memories

When I was a little girl, I remember my mother singing a very lovely song in Hungarian about lilacs. She sang it many times and always there seemed to be a gay and happy feeling as she sang and did her chores. I always thought she must love those flowers very much. As I grew up and received an allowance, I always managed to save some money to buy the first lilacs I saw in the spring. I finished high school during the depression, jobs were scarce and pay very low. But even then Mama got the biggest bunch of lilacs as soon as they were in the flower shops.

Walking in New York several days ago, I saw the lilacs, but was sad that I could no longer see the smile on my mother's face when I walked in the door with her favorite flowers.

May 4, 1979—Reflections

Springtime means flowers starting to bloom, planting gardens, and cleaning up after the winter.

To a housewife it means opening windows to let the balmy breezes into the house, and starting to clean, a monotonous chore, but one which must be done. As I started my usual spring closet cleaning, I found a lamp with a music box that my mother bought for my daughter when she was three months old, it was her first Chanukah present from grandma and grandpa. I wound up the music box and lo and behold it still played "Who's Afraid of the Big Bad Wolf?"

Tears welled in my eyes. I was sad for a while, but then recalling the many happy memories made me feel good.

This also happens when I bring down the boxes with pictures, it usually takes me half a day longer to get finished, but how good it feels to be able to recall happy and sad incidents and say I am so glad I have been able to get older because unfortunately many of my friends were not lucky enough to reach this age. I stopped what I had been doing and sat down to write how I felt.

July 7, 1979

Sitting alone in the apartment, everything is quiet, the radio playing softly. I cannot sleep. It was a good weekend. My daughter, sister, and brother-in-law came to visit to celebrate my birthday. I was sorry my nephew and his family could not make it.

We had dinner at a Hungarian restaurant in Yorkville and listened to Hungarian gypsy music which we all love.

Suddenly, I recalled the times when we were young and went out to dinner with our parents. Always there were the beautiful haunting strains of the gypsy violin and cymbalo. Just thinking of these days gave me a good warm feeling as if someone had draped a warm shawl around me. Memories are so precious, especially as you grow older and are alone. It seems like yesterday that my mother and I looked at an apartment and when she saw the New York skyline—she always loved New York—said, "This is it, let's take it." It was thirty-nine years ago, we were four then, my parents, my husband, and I. Then we were five when our daughter was born. It was a particularly difficult time in my life and yet the happiest when after twelve years and many problems in trying to have a child, I was finally able to. But my mother was very ill and we were told she had only a short time to live.

Mother always said she wanted a granddaughter since my sister had a son, so we were all grateful that she lived to see my daughter.

Shortly after our daughter was born, my parents moved into their own apartment in the same building. My sister and her family were across the street and so my mother's last days were made easier because we were always near her.

As I sit here alone, I am a little sad because my family all live away from New York, but we get together and see each other frequently. Sometimes it seems we see more of each other than families who live close to each other. And so while at times I am a little lonely, I do not dwell on it too much when I think I am fortunate enough to have a good relationship with them.

"Remember": with this word of exhortation, Margaret begins to write of a dream in which she hears the echo of an oft-repeated command: "Practice!" The dream only half-conceals the harshness of her mother's demand upon her. "Practice! Practice!" That was the common battle cry of East European Jewish mothers who wanted their children to march up mountains of respectability and culture, foot soldiers in the ranks led by Heifetz and Elman. Writing of it more than fifty years later, Margaret accepts her mother's claims upon her as natural: she "naturally reminded me of my responsibility." Musical accomplishment has been turned into a normal developmental task, and the child fails. It is a failure both of talent and of will. Of the two hidden charges against her, the badness of her will appears graver than her lack of talent. She kept time, but in the wrong way: not with her fingers on the keyboard, but with her eye on the clock. She preferred reading, a manly activity in traditional Jewish households; little girls who read too much were warned they would end up as old maids. This "bad girl's" lack of musical ability was suspiciously selective: flat notes in general she could recognize; deafness descended upon her only while she was playing the piano.

In the dream, Margaret fulfills her mother's—and her own— wish: she puts on a beautiful performance, "no errors, timing, everything perfect." Upon waking up, she remembers everything, "but I smiled to myself." That apparently illogical "but" is the only acknowledgment of the pain that otherwise makes no noise in this dream of a beautiful concert. And yet the final image sounds a disturbing note: in actuality she goes to the piano not to play it, but to dust it.

Mother, music, and dust appear to be the key images in this passage; each is associated with the master-image of the piano over which Margaret finally gains mastery. But the passage implicitly contains a criticism of this all-too-easy triumph: this is the sort of "beautiful" thing that immediately turns to dust. The dream represents and conceals the resurgence of an unresolved conflict. We may, at this point, guess that Margaret's mother has returned to "remind" her of her "responsibility"; that what she may finally be saying is: "Remember me!" But this is conjecture; the outlines of the conflict are still hidden.

Nearly a month later, in early April, "April Showers" plays upon Margaret's strongly visual imagination and "transport[s]" her to the family dining room in Yorkville. Her imagination moves quickly past the table and the chairs—common things, but Margaret *sees* them, makes them grand and particular—to Mama's sewing machine, a piece of furniture whose symbolic and cultural value in immigrant households rivaled that of the piano; then, landing in front of the player piano, Margaret's daydream becomes populated, becomes charged with a scene that must have been repeated countless times. "Lo and behold," she bursts out, insisting upon the magical power of music—and memory—to bring things to life.

The family used to listen to music together around the player piano. (If she had learned to play properly, would they have had to resort to this automation, programmed by "music rolls"?) Margaret remembers that the members of her family used to sing or whistle in unison with the music—all except her. She never felt that her voice was good enough to join in. Does she feel excluded, blacksheepish? "Those were happy days," she declares. Memory has performed one of its kind offices: whatever pain or conflict she may have felt are purged by the sensation of being reunited with her family, brought together by music.

Margaret's daydream, having coiled itself around the player piano, now makes a marvelous leap to "Fridays" and the "dough of [her mother's] Friday baking" which was "covered by a feather pillow to keep it warm so that it would rise." The aroma and variety of her mother's cakes rise like a rich sensuous legacy in Margaret's imagination; and this evokes her abiding, passionate love: "Nothing but nothing that I eat today tastes half so good as what Mama gave us on Friday afternoon with our milk." Even now, she sees her mother as an abundant giver of milk.

In this passage, Margaret lingers awhile over all that her mother gave her, represents it in a kind of Keatsian rapture, and reveals that it far surpasses everything she has tasted since. Her loss, the impress of it on her prose, is beginning to be felt. Indirectly, writing about this unbidden memory places before Margaret the question which the dream-passage hid from view. Having been given so rich a life by her mother, what did she give in return?

The entry of April 26th answers: lilacs! This is the turning point. It begins with music, which in each of these passages is the Proustian object that leads her back to her mother. In the first passage, all we know of the music is that it is beautiful and perfect; in the second, we hear of operas, the classics, popular tunes. With each entry, the music becomes more specific and more specifically associated with her mother. Here, her mother is singing "a lovely song in Hungarian about lilacs"; and, like lilacs themselves, the song imparts a "happy feeling" to what otherwise might be drab: her mother's doing chores about the house. Now Margaret recaptures the intense happiness she felt as a little girl around her mother, and she feels her generous love overflow in the present as it did in the past. At all times she has brought her mother bouquets of the flower she loved; she does so now by remembering that as a little girl, receiving an allowance, and as a young woman, earning her first salary, she gave her mother "the first" and "biggest bunch" of lilacs that she saw each spring.

Having felt her old happy love for her mother and remembered her loyal spring gift, she makes contact with her grief. The note of sadness has at last entered in. For Margaret, too,

> April is the cruelest month, breeding
> Lilacs out of the dead land, mixing
> Memory and desire

But now the desire to please her mother only distresses her; it's too late for that. Yes, she gave lilacs. Was that enough? Even if they sufficed to repay her mother, to make good the debt, she will nonetheless never again see "the smile on her mother's face when I walk in the door with her favorite flowers." Margaret is no longer smiling, as in the first passage, or in a high state of pleasure, as in the second, after she has tasted her mother's pastries again and been warmed by her mother's sensuous largess. The happiness she associates with her mother's song is gone; she's left with her love, her guilt, and her grief. The loss is, once again, real for her.

The catharsis comes two weeks later while she's engaged in a "monotonous chore" herself. Here, too, housework is charged with meaning; Margaret herself insists on it. To a housewife, she tells us, spring "means flowers starting to bloom . . . it means opening windows to let the balmy breezes into the house." And Margaret, too practiced a lover of language not to use the word wittingly, knows that "balm" is a fragrant thing that has medicinal value, like the memory of lilacs or Hungarian pastries. Spring also "means . . . cleaning up after the winter," which is not quite the same thing as doing a spring cleaning: it tells us that winter has made a mess of things, perhaps by covering them with forgetfulness. For Margaret, cleaning winter's mess specifically means opening her closets and reexamining their contents: "when I bring down the boxes of pictures, it usually takes me half a day longer to get finished, but how good it feels to be able to recall happy and sad incidents." This is a purposeful seeking of reminiscences, or rather objects that will stimulate reminiscence. She handles what she hasn't looked at or touched in a year's time: it is like the anniversary of a death or other landmark event when one rearranges one's memories.

Now she comes upon "a lamp with a music box" that her mother gave to her infant daughter. She winds it up; it plays an old nursery song that scoffs at the fear of death; and again the magic words that announce a sudden apparition spring to her lips: "lo and behold," the nursery song summons her tears. Margaret opens herself fully now to the sorrow towards which she has been moving closer and closer: the death of her mother. Amid images of blossoming, of opening things, she cries. After mourning for her mother anew, she can once again accept things as they are.

Nearly four months after playing the piano in a dream, Margaret comes to the heart of the conflict, and resolves it—for the time being. The death of her mother, like her own birthday, comes round once a year; its anniversary may well have evoked a renewal of grief work. There is a sense of rightness, of completeness, in her thinking of her mother's deathday after celebrating her birthday: the mind moves naturally among natural pairs of opposites. Then, too, Margaret associates her birthday with one or two other things that carry her, in her reverie, to her mother's last days. Her birthday is a time when the scattered members of her family come together. But what is reconstituted, finally, is the scene in the family dining room: Margaret has chosen a restaurant in Yorkville where she and those to whom she is closest can listen to "the Hungarian gypsy music we all love." She recalls dinners out with her parents. The "beautiful haunting strains of the gypsy violin and cymbalo" are the leitmotif which announces the rearrival of her mother. But now, when she comes in, Margaret can work more consciously with the question her mother's reemergence puts to her. For it is her birthday, the day that explicitly raises the theme of gifts; it is a time when we are fully entitled to the gifts we receive, not because we merit them, but because we are alive. For Margaret, *birthday* becomes a configuration of images that calls up the question of what she received from her mother and that simultaneously suggests the terms of her answer to it. Now, at last, she is able to repossess her memory of the real and tremendous gift she gave to her mother, one that was far more acceptable than her annual bunch of lilacs or the perfect rendition of a piece of music. And this gift was made in time! Finally, there were "no errors," the "timing" and "everything" were "perfect." After twelve years of being unable to conceive, Margaret gave birth to a healthy baby. She gave her dying mother what she wanted—a granddaughter; and so she made a gift of life in return. "We were all grateful that she lived to see my daughter." Even here, as she remembers herself as the successful giver, Margaret's thought is of the gratitude she feels.

Between February 27th and July 7th, Margaret has attempted to make restitution—to justify—all that she's been given, and to make peace with her mother's death. Implicit in this sequence of passages is not only the guilt that often afflicts a child at the death of a parent, but also a more specific guilt: Margaret followed more in her father's footsteps, particularly as a young woman. She was a "reader"; she was political, disputatious—qualities that he fostered in her. (She has frequently spoken and written about the way he encouraged her to become an independent, outspoken woman.) Now, she has made the balance right. She has paid homage to her mother's enduring influence not only by keeping the piano with her, even though she cannot play it, but more authentically by her passionate love of music. On the night of her birthday, she has touched on and reintegrated all the elements of her conflict. She has come back into possession of her knowledge that her mother's gift of life was gratuitous, requiring no return gift; that her mother's gift involved not only life but the foundation of a good life, a "fortunate" life filled with "good relationships" and with the kind of richness for which lilacs and gypsy music may stand as the emblems; that even if no return gift was required—for life itself there can be no sufficient repayment—she has nonetheless felt called upon to make one; and she did: she adequately returned her mother's gift by carrying it on and giving birth to a daughter. And because she did, and now reclaims the experience, she can live with her loss and the burden of her gratitude.

She is also better prepared to face what awaits her: for the figure of her mother has a double-aspect and is as much a figure of death as a giver of life. Her birthday is also a day of judgment on which she addresses not only the question of what she gave to her mother but also the question of what meaning she gave to her life. Her mourning, in short, is also a life review.

This may seem paradoxical. The goal of mourning is to restore our sense of innocence and to renew our capacity to be life-glad, so that our involvement with the living takes precedence over our involvement with the dead. The goal of the life review is to prepare us to face death through a reevaluation of our lives, particularly of guilt-laden experiences, and through the discovery of a redemptive "metaphor of self" that is both an emblem of the meaning of our lives and a plausible legacy.

In late life, these two processes are increasingly interwoven:

mourning becomes part of the life review process; the life review becomes part of the process of mourning. For Margaret, or any vigorous older person, the goal towards which each process leads is impossible to attain, unacceptable, and unreal. Mourning can no longer achieve its goal of separating the mourner, as if by a river of forgetfulness, from the great company of the dead; the life review cannot readily help one take leave of the living—not yet. As the two processes become less distinguished by differences of goal, their central similarity becomes apparent: both mourning and the life review make use of recurring reminiscences to manifest and affirm the experience of continuity.

3. *THE VICTIM-SOLDIER*

There is some controversy about whether the life review is "universal' and "normative," as Robert Butler maintains, or whether it is a pathological use of reminiscence made by compulsive people who have been evaluating their experience in a judgmental and obsessive way all their lives. I am of Butler's party, and think that doubt as to the normative character of the life review has arisen in part because we have not had clear descriptions of what actual life reviews look like.

It doesn't help matters that the life review process involves a gradual bringing to light of unconscious or subconscious material: it is therefore by its very nature a hidden process which may assume myriad forms. The life reviews of most older people are not composed of an orderly progression of memories, organized into a coherent narrative. Nor do they remain confined with the boundaries of a recognizable form, such as the journal entry or brief first-person narrative. Life reviews are largely quiltwork affairs, a matter of bits and pieces all stitched together according to a not very readily visible pattern. Or, to use another metaphor, life reviews are dispersed among a great variety of scattered fragments: it is difficult to collect all the pieces of reverie, fantasy and lyric outburst, story-telling and contemplation, and to reconstitute the whole rare amphora they compose.

If life reviews are hidden, fragmentary, and assume many forms, how can we tell when we have come across one?

I would answer: we can discern the life review process in action when we find, amid fragments of reminiscence, a recurring configuration of images that manifests a question and a partial answer to it.

This description implies that the repetition of the configuration of images is the result of a normative problem-solving process, not of a pathological process such as obsessive rumination. Each recurrence may be seen as another attempt to answer the question which the life review manifests and addresses; the process is of necessity repeated until the pieces of the configuration have been put together in a new way, one that provides illumination, wholeness, and harmony.

Irene Salamon's first attempt to review her life in writing clearly exemplifies the proposed description. This life review consists of five apparently unrelated pieces, written over a five-month period. When one reads them closely, it becomes evident that the aim of transforming the figure of the victim into the figure of the soldier governs both her unconscious and her conscious productions, and that the recurring configuration of the victim and the soldier is connected to a search for meaning. The following pieces are presented in the order in which Irene Salamon wrote them:

December 18, 1978—A Walk

The wind howls. I put my scarf over my head and ears, make big steps in my lined boots and march. And to my mind comes another march thirty-two years ago, without warm scarves or lined boots and with a growling stomach. I think back and I wonder: How much can one human endure? It is not a pleasant memory, but now I still enjoy walking in the crisp, fresh air.

January, 1979—A Dream

The rucksack on my back is so heavy. I am very tired, hungry, and thirsty, but I push on, right foot, left foot, I have to reach the top before it gets too dark to see. Every minute feels like an hour. I am weary to the bones. Five more steps and I am there. Four, three, two—I woke up with a scream all prepared, the final step was into nothingness. My heart was pounding and every bone hurts.

Meaning Of Our Generation

I was born shortly before the First World War. For the first four years of my life, my father meant only a picture of a soldier on the dresser. As a teenager in Germany even before the Hitler years, we were growing up with fear and hate and could not understand why. And then we were displaced persons, from riches to rags. There was no loyalty or meaning in our lives. In the DP Camps, we clung to each other, but friendship could not bloom—today you were here, tomorrow gone.

We married in 1948 and came to America. My three children were born here and we tried to live a normal family life. Our nerves were bad and our faith in people was not very strong. The first real joy we experienced was in May, 1948 when the State of Israel became a reality. In order to become a citizen my nephew had to join the war in Korea. As my son Mark grew up there was Vietnam! We did not want him to run away from our adopted country, so he made the decision to join. Do I have to tell you how many sleepless nights and worries we had? Thank G-d, after four years he joined us again—unscathed!

Now that the children are on their own and we retired, we are thankful for every day and enjoy it to the fullest. What meaning our life had—I cannot answer.

I, Judith of Bethulia

I, Judith, was an only child. My father raised me as if I were a son. I can do anything around the many acres of our rich soil. I keep the books, I tend to the house. But now there is a war with the Assyrians and I am not allowed to fight. Everybody says I am beautiful, so I will use my beauty and brains to help win this war. Holofernes, the Assyrian general, is attracted to me. I will invite him to my home outside Bethulia.

After three nights I was able to cut off his head with his own sword. History will show that this war was won by me, a patriotic woman.

May, 1979—Remembering

I had a date with my daughter to go to Lincoln Center to hear *Carmen*. I was pleasantly surprised, how nice she did her long hair and she had a very nice dress on, really looked good. Usually she loves pants. My mind wandered back many years ago: I must have been three or four years old, my older brother was two years older. One evening we wondered why mother closed the door on us. We pestered her and when she finally opened it, our eyes grew big with excitement. Here she was in a gown, her hair done up beautifully and her jewelry shone! The radio was on, and she enjoyed an opera! She believed that clothing is very important to enjoy culture to the fullest.

And here was my daughter doing the same!

In the first piece, a journal entry about an unbidden memory, the figure of the victim of Nazi persecution makes her first fleeting appearance. In the second, a journal entry about a dream, the figure of the Jewish prisoner being marched to her death is fused with that of the marching, battle-fatigued soldier. In the third piece, which is her first deliberate attempt to review her life, the figure of the victim-soldier is replaced by that of the soldier-victim: it is the figure of the soldier as absent family member—and potential victim—that dominates the piece. The shadows of three wars fall across her life, and she structures her life review accordingly: it is divided into three major periods of absence. The First World War figures chiefly as the absence of a soldier-father; the Vietnam War as the absence of a soldier-son; the Holocaust as the absence of meaning. And for her, meaning means other people whom she can trust. She tells us that the Nazis destroyed her faith in people along with her people.

The fourth piece may be described as a "fantasy reminiscence." It is liberating for her to get rid of the sincere narrator who is identical with the author. By assuming the mask of Judith of Bethulia, a beautiful woman and a soldier, she can speak of things that a proper, Orthodox Jewish woman ordinarily keeps well-hidden: sexuality and violence. But the deliberate inauthenticity of the piece permits it. The comic tone, which gives her license, has its source in the flamboyance of two types of stock character: its flaunt is that of the braggart soldier who is every inch the *femme fatale*. And yet it is the comic surface of the piece which indirectly allows her, for the first time, to hint at the horror she lived through: she is letting us in on her own thirst for vengeance. Paradoxically, the piece is what it represents: a high-spirited, audacious act. Irene, her voice ringing with pleasure, becomes Judith in the workshop: usually shy, even timid, she grows powerful and charming as she speaks of cutting off the head of her enemy and saving her people.

The configuration of images that recurs in these four pieces manifests the question that she has chosen to live with consciously. She is asking: What meaning can I find in survivorship? It is important to note that the march she alludes to in the first piece happened "thirty-two years ago," that is, in 1946: she is referring not to the trauma of deportation and imprisonment but to the shock of liberation, of having survived the concentration camp. And the recurring configuration that raises the question also contains the only terms in which it may be answered. The figure of the soldier is telling the victim: you were spared so that you could triumph over those who murdered your people.

"What meaning our life had—I cannot answer": broken in half, that sentence ends her first summary of the significant facts of her life. After answering that question in a fantasy, she goes on, in the fifth piece, to tell a story that embodies the terms of her real triumph over the Nazis and thereby provides her with an emblem of meaning: she has survived to create life and to continue her mother's way of life. The generational continuities she discovers now are female and positive, not male and negative. Looking back earlier at her life, she saw her son, like her father, as an absent soldier. Now she sees that her daughter has turned out to be a woman like her mother—a woman of high culture. Implicit in the story is an assertion of pride and accomplishment: she has been a culture-bearer; she has kept alive and transmitted the beautiful ways of the past.

4. THE CYCLE OF GENERATIONS

The life reviews of Irene Salamon and Margaret Friedman are both conducted under the aegis of a profound and never fully articulated faith: one might call it a belief in the inherent goodness of the cycle of generations. In very different ways, each woman must wrestle with the dead; each must search for an answer to the large question with which the dead leave us: for what have you survived? Each, in answering that question, points to her daughter. Through their daughters, they carry on the gift of their music-loving mothers, the gift of life and of a particular way of life. But they do not want to attach their daughters to the past. Rather, their relationships with their daughters, with whom they are close, help free them from the past so that they may live lives that are open to the future. By bridging the generations, by taking their place in the cycle of generations, they play a real, infinitesimal, age-old role in sustaining human life on the earth and in handing down their culture's version of it. This gives them a firm place to stand in the present as they feel the presence of death in their past and their future.

The life review process is an ongoing one. Peace may be won, but it is usually something like a truce between renewed outbreaks of conflict. Now, in their third year of meeting together, the people in the Astoria Workshop have undertaken a year-long "autobiography project." Rather than feel they have exhausted that subject during the course of the "journal project" and the subsequent "reverie project," they feel that the life review pieces they previously wrote have prepared them to reconsider their entire life-histories and to write book-length narratives.

Irene calls her autobiography *A Kaleidoscope of My Life*. In her chapters on adolescence and young adulthood, she speaks in detail of the persecution that she and her family suffered before the war and of the hardships they endured after it. Of her four years in German concentration camps she has refused to write, but she has begun to talk about those years in the workshop. Writing her autobiography, in addition to enabling her to venture onto terrain that was once off-limits, has given her a chance to survey her life once again, not only to document it, but to discover where the meaning is hidden. Now, what lay beyond her grasp is obvious to her: she recovers and consciously possesses the "answer" to which the earlier life review pointed but could not yet utter directly. How passionately she proclaims it now! Coming back to the birth of her daughter, she retells the story as the rebirth of meaning in her life:

> Through June and July, I was mostly in bed and on July 8, 1949, our Pearl was born. Amazing how such an event can change your whole life. A new leaf on a nearly dried-out tree! Life had meaning again and was worth fighting for. My husband and I promised each other to do everything possible, so that she would grow up free in America and be whatever she wanted to be with G-d's help. There was no place for a crib, so we opened a drawer and that was her bed.

The Passion of Recollection

Barbara Baracks

Mors auren vellens, "vivite," ait, "venio."
Here's Death twitching my ear, "Live," says he,
"for I'm coming."—from "Dancing-Girl of Syria"
("Copa Surisca")
Tradition attributes this poem to Virgil

We are sitting in a circle in a carpeted room. To one side is a coffee urn and what's left of the cake. In the middle of the floor is a tape recorder. Sonya, who recently emigrated here from the Soviet Union, occasionally jokes about my selling the tapes to the KGB. But for the most part, after meeting weekly for two months, everyone's become pretty good at ignoring the machine.

Aiesha, eighty-two-years old, is describing becoming old: "This state of mind comes gradually. And because this comes gradually, you're accustomed to it. Last year I was in Freeport, I was helping a friend of mine. And every morning there is a point where the boats come in. Every morning to this point and back, I can make it, four miles a day. I was very satisfied. I believe this is a normal thing. But I will go to Freeport next week, and I will try to make the same thing, to make four miles. I am not sure of that. If I make the half of that I will be satisfied. I will tell you: 'Is not bad.' I cannot explain this medically or scientifically. But there is a state of our brain which tells you: Be satisfied. . . . Physical suffering is a terrible life, especially when you are alone and you know that there is no health. I believe there is more courage to suffer. To throw yourself out of the window, it's hard to do—but this is five seconds."

Soon after Aiesha spoke, Lisette, who also is eighty-two, began weeping, because, she said, she was not kind to her sister, who died twelve years ago. She has told this to the group many times. "I didn't talk to her for a long time before she died, and I heard when she was dying she cried for me—"

Sonya, in her seventies, gently interrupted: "I want to tell you a story, a funny story."

We are involved in a reminiscence workshop, and we are newcomers to what we're doing. Because this group consists of particularly old people, there is difficulty, and tenderness, and illumination in the ways people in the group reach out not just to their individual pasts, but to each other sitting in the room together.

Kitty Urquhart, a social worker, is coleading this group with me. Her extraordinary ability to sense and draw out feelings in the group has been a rare lesson to me with all my impatience. This impatience, a journalistic bias towards facts rather than feelings, has gotten in my way, especially the first few times the group met. A lot has happened in a short period of time. After eight meetings—midpoint in the group's fifteen-week lifespan—I can offer documentation and some insights along the way on what the group and I are beginning to discover.

I am one of several writers, funded by CETA through the Cultural Council Foundation, who are working with the Artists & Elders Project. Organized by Teachers & Writers Collaborative in March, 1979, the project conducts workshops for older adults in a wide variety of settings, including union halls, libraries, senior centers, and nursing homes. This, my first assignment, is taking place at the Service Program for Older People (SPOP), a not-for-profit social agency in Manhattan which counsels older people with psychological and/or physical problems. Caseworkers at SPOP suggested clients who might be interested in the project, and the agency has donated space and resources and given Kitty time for the group meetings.

The group is not a large one. Some people drop in and out, but three women are regulars every week: Sonya, in love with America, fiercely independent, optimistic, sympathetic; Lisette, whose reading of pop psychology preens the plumage of her neuroses, lately beginning to trust her own perception of things; Aiesha, frail, passionate, intelligent, coy—a morbid and thoughtful philosopher. Some people don't come every time because their physical disabilities are a great obstacle to travel, even with the assistance I'm willing to provide with a taxi ride. Others don't come at all because they see what we're doing as strange, frightening, confusing. Or boring. There is no easy label to put on the kind of talking the group does. It isn't strictly a social group, like the "Friday group" that meets at

SPOP. Nor is it oral history in the more directly documentary tradition of Studs Terkel.

I didn't know that when the group first met. I was eager for results and came armed with a selection of ready-made topics for recollection. I thought we would concentrate on specific themes— work, love relationships, childhood, etc.—with the narrowness of purpose of so many bees swarming out for the pollen. We couldn't just sit around and talk, this was supposed to be *work*—right? My anxiousness was quickly communicated, and the results were brittle, like sitting down and trying to write without giving your mind a little breathing space to ramble along and talk to itself, warm up.

By the third meeting it looked like the whole project had fallen apart. From my notes, taken from listening to the tapes at home:

We then discussed Aiesha's forty-year sojourn in Egypt. She lived in Cairo. Unfortunately we didn't get much further than that. Lisette brought out a picture of her son, and we got onto the subject of children instead. Aiesha was talking about China, all the while Lisette was showing me the picture of her son. It's frustrating listening to the tape of Lisette plunging in as soon as Aiesha starts saying something on her own. When Aiesha once again began talking about being a nurse in Cairo, Lisette showed me a picture of herself. I'm madder now than I was then about it! Then she brought out a picture of her daughter. Then we got onto the delicate subject of whether or not to have kids. I wanted to inquire into Aiesha's lack of kids, but in order not to be tactless about it, I talked about the probability that I may well never have children. And lo and behold, Lisette came in with a story about the king of Spain.

It was as if we were locked up in separate boxes lying side by side. We remained painfully isolated people rehearsing pain, both past and present, aware that no one really was listening to anyone else. "The immobility of the things that surround us," Proust called it. "Things" are what we still were to each other.

It was then, supersaturated with formulae, that we—or rather Aiesha—broke through. She began talking about what really was on her mind, something that had happened just the other day. From my notes:

Aiesha was translating for a man with an old Russian mother. (It seems that though the mother speaks Russian the son does not, and they can't communicate with each other without a translator.) He had put his mother in a home, a "good" one—since he had money—in the Bronx. The son had called Aiesha because he'd written to the home three times without getting an answer. Aiesha went up to the home with a letter for the mother from her son. "This is Mother's Day," he wrote. "Tell my mother my best regards. We put her photo on the table on Mother's Day and eat around the photo." The mother, Aiesha found, was totally senile. She didn't remember anything, not even that she had a son. "She didn't remember," Aiesha said. "She asked, 'Who is Yanid?' and then she started to cry, to take her to the children, she wanted to be out of this house. It was pathetic. The problem is that she is in good health except her head." And now Aiesha came to her point. "I think," Aiesha continued, "there must be a law. When you come to certain age, when you have this kind of case, make an injection and finish with this kind of thing. . . . I certainly, after a year or two, when I am not able, I will make an injection and I will be finished, certain."

Thanks to Aiesha's introduction of death and dying to the conversation, everyone became alive again. Lisette in particular was furious at the idea of euthanasia, especially when Aiesha went on and said that if old people weren't willing to kill themselves, then a commission of doctors should decide for them. The great taboo about death had been violated, and the great thaw had begun.

The subject of death and dying came up, after that, again and again, in the shape of losses of friends, family, powers of mind and body. It was invigorating. People began speaking with detailed commitment about the past and present. We began to like each other. (We decided to take a couple of trips outside the group meetings—one to the Cloisters, and one to the Museum of Natural History's Pompeii exhibit.) Memories became resonant, and the grappling hook of everyday experience began stirring up all kinds of strange material from the past: mud and debris, odd fishes, jokes, governesses, terrible corpses, childhood sweethearts.

We have begun to talk about relative degrees of loneliness. Sonya on her husband's cancer: "He couldn't work and he was in bed four months. He suffered so. He told me, 'If there wouldn't be gossip about you I would make suicide. I would throw myself from the fifth floor.' He loved me very much and he was a very good man. So when he died I didn't cry. He suffered. In three days I went back to work." Kitty remarked that Sonya had said her husband was

devoted to her. "How," Kitty asked, "did you feel about him?"
"He loved me," Sonya said, "more than I loved him."

Lisette on her escape from her family's strict French-Algerian
household: "I didn't take a step outside unless my mother was with
me, from when I was twelve years old until I was about twenty-one.
I would marry anybody. He asked for my hand, he was an American
soldier. He was ugly, he was terrible, and he was poor. I was very
disgusted, I could not kiss him, but I said I will, and I married
him."

Sonya has a job helping people in a nursing home. She described
it: "I know a lovely woman, she plays accordian. She told me, 'I am
never lonely.' She washes the windows in the room. Always she
do something. What a wonderful woman. Ninety-two and three
months. . . . She was a dressmaker for the best artist in New York.
She had a beauty salon, she was very rich. What else? She was a
painter, she has her pictures on the wall. I love her very much. Her
husband died three years ago and now because she fell she cannot
walk, she is in a wheelchair. But she wants to go to the concert. . . . All day she does something. . . . You know, I became a
philosopher in this nursing home. Because so many people, they
were long ago. One was a famous architect, his pictures are in the
room, and now he is nothing. We have one Hungarian diplomat
here—and now he's nothing. He doesn't understand anything. So
you have to be a philosopher, because—"

Aiesha interrupted here: "So you have to make an injection and
make it go away."

Sonya: "Not so easy. He wanted it, the former architect, he
wanted to make suicide. But unfortunately they saved him."

Aiesha: "And I don't understand why they saved him."

Sonya: "I thought much time about that, even when I was young.
Such people have not to live, but if they say it be a rule, they will
begin to kill healthy people."

Aiesha: "We have a limit of time. We have a vegetable, a senile
vegetable, for two years. It's finished!"

Aiesha later continued: "Most people—how sick you are you
never believe. I tell you, I remember this boy, it was in the Russian
Revolution. He was only twenty years old. And I took him from the
battlefield, he had his belly open. Is nothing there, maybe some in-
testine. Everything was out, this was an explosive thing. Then we
come to the battlefield, you know they took the dead, the critically
wounded. He was a critical case, there was nothing to do. And we

put him in the train. When we took him on the train, his bed was near the passage where I was coming and going, making injections, giving some drinks or some pills. Every time where I pass he was grabbing me—where he could reach, he couldn't talk properly. He was speaking to me, saying, 'Nurse, I will not die, I will not die.' He was a beautiful boy, maybe twenty-one, I was twenty-one too. He was always grabbing me, by my shirt, hold me, 'I will not die—' ''

Sonya interrupted: "I knew a man, it was at a resort. When he understood he had cancer, he cut his throat."

Lisette: "What happened to that boy?"

Aiesha finished: "I was always saying, 'Misha, no. Never, never.' But he died. When I brought him he was dead. I knew he would not come to the hospital, I was sure of that. I didn't want to tell him. He had plenty of life, plenty willing to live, to enjoy. He was grabbing me: 'Nurse, nurse.' ''

And so, back to the present. Sonya said: "I have an ulcer, but we live together in peace."

Aiesha: "When you're alone, how can you be optimistic? How normal are you if you stay alone? There is a certain decline in your mind—"

Sonya: "Loneliness is a very good thing if you have a friend to tell about your loneliness."

Already looming over us is the group's ending. We have our own momentum now—and stopping after fifteen weeks feels to me like flying a 747 from New York to Philadelphia. Why not go all the way to the Antipodes while we're at it? It's hard for me to think of ending the group, and for some of these people, who have fewer distractions and parallel projects than I, it may be harder.

But we haven't discussed continuing the group. No one has brought it up. There remain indirectly stated suspicions and testing. Recently Sonya said: "I told my son, 'Now I go to a group. It seems to me I am a psychology rabbit.' ''

Being a guinea pig, the object of someone else's manipulation—it's a reasonable fear. Kitty and I are strangers bearing gifts. In writing this, I keep testing my own feelings toward the group. Nicole, whose severe arthritis makes it hard for her to go anywhere, once said, "I always go up to Columbia and sit to see all the young people around."

But it was cheerful, people-loving Sonya who, in reply, drew the line: "Among young people I'm old, I'm not beautiful. I think the young people and the old people, they should be separate."

A caste system of generations allows, under usual circumstances, only the most perfunctory exchange. Sonya described the realities very well: "Sometimes if a woman lives all her life, she has everything, she is still depressed. In Russia is very good proverb: 'From fat is crazy.' She is excited and becomes mad. That's true. Because in Russia, for example, if, in my age, I have to take care of four children—grandchildren, for example—because my children work. And I have to prepare for them the food but I have to go stand in line. And when I will stand three hours in line I will receive meat or butter, I will come and I will be lucky, very happy. But if I will wake up and I will have everything and I am alone—so I will be depressed."

Sonya's son lives in this country also, but not near her. How she dealt with this became clear when Aiesha asked her why she went to work (first as a volunteer, later as a paid employee) in a nursing home. Sonya answered: "I have a disaster. When my grandson died, I wanted to be busy. Because I thought I had no right to live. So I wanted to be useful. I went to the nursing home . . . I wanted to justify my existence."

Aiesha listened with intense interest to Sonya's long descriptions of her work in the nursing home. Yet in previous weeks Aiesha had sourly complained that even though she was retired, people kept calling on her for medical services. (A few weeks ago a neighbor who had just collapsed with a stroke in a grocery store called Aiesha instead of an ambulance!) Finally, unable to contain herself, Aiesha began firing questions at Sonya: Why was she working there? Wasn't she a professional pianist? And finally: Where is this nursing home?

Snug Harbor:
Workshops at the National
Maritime Union

Dale Worsley

1. FINDING THE GOAL

When I was hired by CETA to work as a fiction writer in the community, I asked to be placed in a job with the elderly because they would be likely to tell interesting stories. Eventually I was assigned to work with retired seamen at the National Maritime Union (through the Artists and Elders Project). My stars were very good. Who could possibly tell more stories than seamen? I pictured myself sitting around a wharf amidst a group with tattooed skin, sailor's caps and pipes (upon which they perhaps tooted). Palm trees swayed in the breeze and the gulls cried as they followed ships out in the harbor.

Later, in April 1979, I was walking through the grimmer reality of 17th Street in Manhattan toward the union building, to start the project. As I approached, I realized the only really substantial thing I knew about seamen was what I recalled from literature—very little more than the fantasy I'd painted originally. What I knew about maritime unions had filtered down to me when I lived landlocked in the south, where unions are suspect and maritime unions in particular are feared for their reputed violence. At the entrance to the building, where men and women without tattoos or caps were going in, I panicked a little.

Inside I passed a security guard and well-equipped gymnasium, took the elevator up to Dan Molloy's office (in Personal Services).

We discussed the upcoming workshops, then went into the cafeteria to talk more and meet some of the pensioners who'd shown interest. In the food line I was introduced to a bright, very well-dressed man in his sixties named Bill Gavin. In desperation I said, "I don't know anything about the merchant marine, or life at sea."

"That's all right," he said. "What do you want to know?"

His answer relieved my intense apprehension, but I didn't know yet what I wanted to know. I asked him what he'd done as a sailor, and he explained he had been an oiler. I didn't know what an oiler was and was too embarrassed to ask. I asked him instead when he first sailed, and if that was still the proper word, *sail*.

"I first sailed out of Fort Williams, Ontario, back in the thirties," he said. "I'd been bumming around with a friend of mine. . ."

By the time we paid the cashier at the end of the food line, I realized I could talk with Bill Gavin. For one thing, I'd bummed around a few years back myself, and we were able to compare notes about that. For another, Bill was very patient by nature. He was interested in taking the time to explain the particulars of seamanship to me. My mind was a blank slate. There would be no danger of telling me anything I already knew, and I had none of the prejudices a more informed man might have had. We had lunch with the others and talked more, and I began to look on Bill as a sort of treasure, a man incredibly rich with stories and the intelligence to put them in historical perspective. The way the workshops were to shape up, I was to meet with any interested men two hours every Wednesday afternoon for at least ten sessions. I practically begged Bill to come to them. He said he would come back next week, a bit amused at my naiveté.

Bill indeed came back the following week, and for all the sessions after that. He more or less guided me into the unknown world of seamen. A total of fifteen other men tried the workshops in the TV lounge of the union building. Most came in for one or two sessions and drifted on, but five became regulars. We got to know each other well, over what turned out to be sixteen workshops. A kind of front-porch atmosphere evolved, with plenty of kidding around and, occasionally, serious personal talk.

The five regulars were a diverse bunch: a Black from Miami, a Hispanic from Panama, a Pole from Boston, a Hispanic from Brooklyn (who wasn't actually retired) and Bill, a WASP from Canada. I felt privileged to be with this crew of men, not only because they opened up to an outsider like me, but because I was party to such a successfully integrated group of people. This successful blending of diverse backgrounds was not a coincidence, I discovered. A watchword in the formation of the NMU back in 1937 had been "Black and White Together," and therein lay the original strength of the union that was now manifest in our group.

Before I met them, I'd conceived of my job with these men in terms of a creative writing workshop. I'd thought we would extend into modern times the rich history of the literature of the sea from the point of view of the ordinary "jack." When I got to know them, it became clear the best tack for this would be to record their stories. Whereas they were quite comfortable speaking, most would have balked at a proposal to write. Some, in fact, claimed they couldn't write. Consequently, the workshops became a kind of oral history project.

As the sessions progressed, I became more educated about the concerns of seamen. I discovered what an "oiler" was and what that meant in relation to the other jobs on a ship. I satisfied my curiosity about the differences between sailing ships and modern shipping. I soon knew enough to direct the conversations and stories to make sure we probed comprehensively all the aspects of their lives at sea. I did this by introducing topics at the beginning of each session, making sure each man had a chance to speak on them, and interjecting whenever anyone seemed in danger of sailing too far off course. The group thus evolved a goal, which was to create a "book" and make it as thorough as possible. Throughout the sessions, the fact of my being a tabula rasa provided a fruitful dynamic. They supplied the material and trusted my ability to see it was organized to its best advantage.

Though a book became our final goal, many by-products were discovered along the way. It was an amazing thing to blow the fog away from certain memories, for one. It was also important to air beliefs as men and as seamen. Many other purposes were served, mostly ones that will always attend the efforts of a team working toward a goal. In the end, the book itself emerged. We were successful. As far as extending the literature of the sea into modern times, I don't know if that is what we accomplished. It doesn't matter. I wish a proverb were handy, one about setting out to do one thing and, once finished, finding out you've done another more to the point.

2. PROBLEMS

Naturally, during the course of the workshops, certain problems had to be resolved. The first one came up before I was involved. When Dan Malloy tried to get a program for pensioners off the ground a year before, the union officials were reluctant to allow space for them to meet. Their hesitations stemmed from an incident in Puerto Rico where pensioners had been allowed to meet and had organized a firebrand rebellion against some of the current policies of the union. The officials in New York didn't want any such dissension here. Eventually they softened their position and provided space for the workshops, and fortunately, for me as well as them, though perhaps for different reasons, the men didn't become activists.

The second problem that arose was to find the best method to use in conducting the workshops. The evolution of the oral history idea has been mentioned. The way it came about was largely the result of the first official meeting with the pensioners. There were eight in all. Half were willing to write, but no one was enthusiastic about putting pen to paper. I had a tape recorder there for that eventuality. I turned it on and tried to induce one man at a time to speak on a specific topic. The topic, which I pulled out of a hat, was "emergencies aboard ship." A couple of the men spoke stiffly about this. This route was too uncomfortable to be viable, so I turned the tape recorder off and broke out in a cold sweat about what to do next. The men were looking to me for guidance, and I had none. To aggravate the situation, a very strange and blindly egotistical man was beginning to filibuster the session with a recitation of transcendental poetry that no one wanted to hear and a lecture on reincarnation that struck us as complete balderdash. I didn't know what to do to make the situation work, but I knew that if this man kept talking, the workshops were doomed. I spoke firmly to him and managed to damp his fires momentarily. At that point a couple of the men started discussing the difference between passenger ships and cargo ships. The discussion got very lively. I furtively turned on the tape recorder. Later I played back part of the tape for them, and we all realized it was possible simply to converse and be recorded. Our basic procedure was thus achieved, but it was nip and tuck in there for a while.

The third major problem that came up relates to the one of the egotist, whose obsessions threatened to destroy the workshops. It is a demon with many heads. It involves the wholeness of the group itself versus the needs of individuals. The transcendental poet was clearly an anomaly for whom we could do no good and who could only sabotage the group's delicate machinery. Though he came back a couple more times, I always let him know he was getting out of hand firmly enough so that he finally stopped coming. Other cases aren't so clear. Notably, one of the five regulars took medication that made him a speed rapper. If he had too much rope, he'd turn you into a psychiatrist with his paranoid, depressed monologues. Through the willingness of the other men to extend him sympathy, however, and the deft orchestration of time allotted to each man to speak his mind, we were successful in both doing him some thera- peutic good and evoking comments from him that were apropos of the book. At various times the quirks of other personalities also threatened our progress, but never so much that a comment from me or a change of subject and perspective by one of the other men couldn't prevent a disaster.

The last hurdle of any consequence faced by the workshop was one that recalls the first. Seamen tend to be outspoken men. If they weren't, they'd have no union and they'd still be working under a lash of one kind or another. These particular seamen struggled forty-three years ago against practically insuperable odds to form a union that served them decently. They are the founders of the NMU. They have kept their fingers firmly pressed to its pulse throughout its existence, and they have things to say about it now that seem extremely controversial. Besides their opinion of certain union matters, they have led lives that exposed them to many of the seamier phenomena of the world, and they don't hesitate to describe them in picturesque detail. These two areas of controversy pre- sented problems. If we had been producing the book independently of the union, we'd have been free to say anything we wanted. Because it was a book cosponsored by the union, however, too much emphasis on decadence and too harsh a criticism of the union were intolerable. To pick our way through this thicket, I devised a procedure. After the material had been recorded, transcribed, edited, corrected by the men, and approved by them (which in itself eliminated some of the controversial statements), I took it to Dan Molloy and asked him to redline anything that he had doubts about. He generously performed this unpleasant task and returned the stories to me. I then showed the men the areas he indicated, and they ruled whether to include them despite Dan's doubts. Almost always they went along with Dan and felt the material was not important enough to fight over. They generally had the opinion it was exaggerated and would taint the rest of the book anyway. A very real conflict was thus averted and the book's life was assured without any loss of integrity.

3. SEAMEN

Having walked into the NMU building completely ignorant of both conducting workshops with the elderly and of the merchant marine, then having held sixteen sessions with articulate retired seamen, I came out with a more informed view of both matters. It's difficult to talk about them separately, however. At every juncture I saw that as individuals, as elders, and as a group, the men were seamen and spoke as seamen. Though most of them will never sail again, and though they live days completely filled with the activities of stationary men, they have the identities of seamen. Often in our meetings the men would try and cajole me into becoming a seaman. They wanted me to understand what it was like. They went to great lengths to illustrate, using their lives as examples. As a group, they understood each other clearly because they had common experiences and spoke a common jargon. I had the feeling the workshops were only a small extension of the rag chewing that might occur in the forecastle.

One of the first things that defined this group as a crew of seamen was the integration I described above. These men united in the thirties in a terrible struggle against powerful enemies to gain decent wages, living conditions fit for a human, and a new status in the world—one raised above the criminal, second-class status accorded seamen earlier.

"In order to become a merchant marine fifty years ago, you had to be rough. There was no such thing as a sissy seaman. This union was built by criminals. By hoodlums. Let's face it. This union was built by men. You had to have guts to build this union in those times. Not only the union, but to go on ships."—Jose Valverde

"There was a whole new education of the crew that went along with this unionism. There were a lot of books and literature brought on the ships . . . . I didn't want anything to do with tattoos. . . . We were going to be a new generation."—Bill Gavin

Hardly had these young men beat poverty, formed a union and begun their education as a new breed of laborer, when the sea-lanes became America's "first front line" in the Second World War. Eisenhower dubbed the merchant marine the "fourth arm," and these seamen indeed had to fight like soldiers. They suffered submarine, battleship, and air attacks in seas around the world, carrying eighty percent of the supplies for the Allied effort and a great majority of America's seven million troops. Phil Valdez was torpedoed twice the same Easter Sunday morning in the Caribbean. He and Tony Zajkowski made the dangerous Murmansk runs through the Arctic Ocean. They are all proud of their record, but feel they didn't reap the benefits they deserved when the fighting stopped. Though the merchant marine lost more men, proportionately, than any branch of the service, they are not recognized as veterans.

"I was in one of the first convoys to Murmansk, in February, right after we declared war. Thirty-eight ships we lost. Eight returned. Absolutely no protection from the Luftwaffe, the wolfpack submarines, the German navy. We lost the British battle cruiser *Trinidad* on the way over, the *Edinburg* on the way back. We carried 5,000 tons of TNT. We were on the outside, so in case we were hit we wouldn't blow the whole convoy. . . ."—Tony Zajkowski
"There were no labels on the torpedoes saying, 'we're for so-and-so.' They hit the vessel and everybody went. Some survived and some didn't. . . . We had military orders, military escorts. We passed ammunition. We fired guns. We got a lot of praise. . . ."—Phil Valdez
"I was in the Pacific, where the Japanese were attacking with kamikaze pilots, in a tanker ship. You've got no chance on there. Yet they don't recognize you as a veteran."—Jose Valverde

There are still appeals being made to Congress to rectify this situation, and it's still possible these men will be awarded benefits thirty-five years later. Either way, there's no disputing the value of their harsh and idealistic experience, which fomented hundreds of stories, only a fraction of which we had time to share.
The status of seamen has always risen and fallen with the tides of economic, political, and military history. Following the Second World War, it hit low tide on every count. The shipping industry declined when practically every other industry boomed. The unions were compelled to clear up their uneasy ties with communist organi-

zations to survive the postwar red-baiting that flared up in this country. As a result, internal union operations were chaotic and uncertain. The Liberty ships that had provided work for so many sailors were now being torched for scrap. In addition to this, the new ships that were eventually produced were more mechanized. Crew complements declined, jobs became more boring, and the traditional skills of seamen began to vanish—just as living conditions on board were reaching practically luxurious levels. Issues of all sorts were no longer cut and dried. To survive, seamen had to adapt. It was another test of their resilience and intelligence that molded their identities.

"The place I remember most is Cuba."—Jose Valverde

"Havana, of course, was the greatest port of them all."—Bill Gavin

"Everything went."—Jose Sanabia

"With ten dollars, you could have a beautiful time in Havana. It was like a paradise."—Jose Valverde

"It was a paradise."—Jose Sanabia

"There was a bar there called Sloppy Joe's. A Coca-Cola cost more than a whole bottle of rum. It was a meeting place. It looked like an ordinary bar, but it had more young women there than we had men."—Phil Valdez

"The police were all racketeers in Havana."—Bill Gavin

"I won't forget Barranquilla, Colombia, with the girls out in the moonlight. Young girls . . . you're dancing and you're drinking . . . the atmosphere."—Tony Zajkowski

"The average seaman tries to make up in port for what he missed doing from the last port he was in. I used to be an alcoholic. I used to say, 'If I die, I die with it in *me*, not in the bottle.'"—Phil Valdez

"If I kept going to sea, I'd be dead within a year. . . I was in Hudson & Jay Hospital. The doctor says, 'You've got alcoholic neuritis in your ankles. If you don't stop drinking and start eating, you're going to die of total paralysis. This is going to creep up your body. . . ' I still have a little limp. I never told my wife. I told her my other wife used to have a chain on my leg."—Tony Zajkowski

"The thing about drinking or not drinking is there comes a time in your life . . . it doesn't matter where you are . . . when you've got to think to yourself, 'Am I going to grow up? Or am I going to keep on the same road that I'm going?' I can't tell you what to do. You have to say this to yourself."—Bill Gavin

"I always tried to improve what I was doing, to make it easier for tomorrow. That was my plan. Probably something will come up in the future and you will change and do something else, but you still try to make improvements. You still try to improve M-E."—Phil Valdez

"They're running these big ships with what, five men on a crew? When I was sailing we had a complement of thirty-seven. They were the old up-and-down jobs. With these turboelectric synchronizers you're just a bookkeeper."—Tony Zajkowski

"I was on a ship called the Marine Dow Chem. We used to come out of Freeport, Texas, with thirty-two different kinds of chemicals in one load . . . . After the war, as years went on, they were getting more complicated all the time . . . . It was very difficult for the company and the workers to keep up to what danger and what threat really went on . . . . Until something happened, you wouldn't know how safe it was."—Bill Gavin

"I'm a sailor. I've been on deck all my life. The way it is today, you get aboard ship and you have a man and he calls himself an AB but he can't splice or steer. He can't go aloft. We had one kid who was an AB. They sent him up on the mast to secure the jumbo boom, to put the pin in the thing and put the collar around it. He froze up there. He actually froze. We had to go up and get the bastard."—Jose Sanabia

When a man chooses to become a seaman, he accepts certain realities that few other men have to contend with. His job is lonely, transitory, devoid of lasting friendships. Sustaining a family or a successful romance is extremely difficult. Older seamen assumed when they went to sea that they would have no control over the forces that directed and often oppressed their lives. Tradition reinforced alcoholism, and vices were at their fingertips (or fully in their hands) at every port. Survival in the teeth of these conditions is practically a miracle. It is a tribute to the power of their will that these men not only survived but braced their strengths and shaped their lives to appreciate and participate creatively in the times now at hand.

These men are survivors. Their mettle has been tested. They are equipped to deal with the world. Now they must deal with retirement. Some are handling it well, fitting in comfortably to the niches our culture offers the elderly. Others have encountered even more loneliness than at sea and are finding this their greatest test. Our workshops relieved that loneliness for a brief spell, and, for most who participated, accomplished much more. The conversations grew into stories, and the stories began to uncover long hidden memories. With the ordering of these memories, a history began to take shape, a history full of fact, fiction, myth, parable and joke, a history that conveyed a meaning. And the meaning, the peculiar and valuable meaning of life as a seaman, once communicated, became a huge affirmation.

"Tell about your chicken farm."

"I never had no chicken farm."

"Who was I talking to?"

"A lot of people had chicken farms."

"You figure you get two chickens and one rooster and the next thing you know is, you got a thousand chickens."

"We used to have a saying, 'red beans and rice.' Retire down to Cuba and eat red beans and rice."

"New Orleans is the red beans and rice place."

"Who was it used to talk about his brooders and all that?"

"There were a lot of people had chicken farms. Seamen are always dreaming and talking about what they're going to do when they retire. When I was sailing into Houston, the night engineers used to come on board and come down into the engine room and be talking about the place they either had or were going to get up in Arkansas. It was always in Arkansas. And they were either going to grow chickens or pigs or strawberries. I don't know why. It was always one of those three. They talked about the nice spring water, the good land in the country that wouldn't cost you too much. This was their dream."

"They called it Snug Harbor."—Bill Gavin and Tony Zajkowski

A Stage for Memory:
Living History Plays by Older Adults

Susan Perlstein

1. A HISTORY OF THE HODSON DRAMA GROUP

On Sunday, June 10, 1979, the Hodson Senior Center Drama Group performed an original play, *Three Generations*, in the South Bronx Center auditorium. Fourteen older women—singing, dancing, and acting—dramatized the ways in which family life had changed over the past seventy-five years. Like ancient balladeers, they wanted to transmit to friends, neighbors, and relatives their collective odyssey. Those who came to see them bear witness ranged in age from three to ninety. Children watched their grandmothers, daughters and sons saw their mothers in a new light. From reminiscing, life review, and oral histories, the Hodson Drama Group created a play that validated the life experience of older adults. The group entertained, educated, and enriched the lives of the people in its community.

How did Hodson Drama Group develop the "living history play"? The process slowly evolved over the past three years. The group met weekly for two-hour workshop sessions in which they shared stories, developed dance and theater skills, put together plays, and rehearsed them.[1] They began as an exercise/dance class. At the completion of the first exercise/dance workshop series, the group gave an open performance for Center members. Everyone was nervous, never having performed before, but felt it was important to share with others what they had learned about care for the body and creative expression through movement. In November 1977, thirty-five seniors performed dance exercises and dance improvisations called "Walking Tall." To everyone's delight and amazement, the open workshop was greatly appreciated, and the group members felt a new confidence in themselves and a desire to move on.

Shortly after the first performance, one of the key members of the group died. As often happens, the unexpected influenced the group's direction. Feeling the loss of Adela, people in the group remembered her interest in making theater part of the Center, and they wished to incorporate drama as part of the workshop. The group continued as a drama group and later dedicated the first play to her.

The play came out of a growing desire to get to know more about the individuals in the group. Questions were asked such as: "Where did you come from?" "What kind of work did you do?" "How did you come to live in the Bronx?" From these questions, we evolved *A Slice of Our Lives*, or what might be called the Hodson version of *Roots*. Interestingly, the group represented a cross-section of the Center membership, so the stories selected and used in the play represented the Center's population. In the prologue, each performer described where she was born and raised. Act I, "The Beginnings," recounted three stories. The first was about growing up in a fishing village on the island of St. Croix. The second showed a sharecropper family in South Carolina. The third dealt with a young girl's journey north to New York City from Montgomery, Alabama to visit her merchant marine father. Act II brought things back home to the Hodson Senior Center and presented the monthly birthday party. People looked back at where they had come from and looked forward to engaging in new activities at the Center.

A sense of self-awareness and excitement grew as a result of sharing life experiences with others. It was a new kind of theater, one that spoke directly to the lives of the audience. When *A Slice of Our Lives* played at Hodson Center, members of the audience said, "It was the best show I've ever seen," and insisted the Hodson Drama Group perform the play for their friends at other centers. So, they took the show on the road and in the spring of 1978, brought it to several senior centers in the neighborhood. Eventually they became featured performers at "A Life Review Festival in Celebration of Aging" held at Wave Hill Center in the Bronx. Bus loads of seniors from centers throughout the borough came to see the show and were appreciative, cheering the performers and asking how they could start their own Living History Theater group. It wasn't long before the New York City Department on Aging acknowledged the group's work with an award for outstanding community service.

New kinds of problems were generated from this modest success.

When the group began again in September 1978, they set up a schedule in which they tried to anticipate problems. For example, the group decided to be open to new members during the exploratory workshops. In addition, each person had to commit herself through the performance period, which usually lasted four months. People were free to leave and come back into the group at the start of a new series. If a member decided to leave, she gave her reasons and expressed her long-range interest in the group. This policy reinforced each member's sense of collective responsibility; it was important in planning ahead, since over forty people had participated at different times.

The group decided to try to create two shows a year—a holiday celebration and a living history play, both of which would reflect the life experience of the group's members. The 1978 holiday show was called *Seasons Greetings*. This play gathered together two large, poor families; its scenes showed the traditional food preparations, holiday decorating, and the children's hour. At this juncture, the men became performance-shy and dropped out. Though the men enjoyed telling their tales, acting was a step they were not anxious to take. It was easier for women to share intimate stories and real feelings about the main events in their life. The living history play, *Three Generations*, told about the changing role of the family from the women's point of view. In the spring of 1979, after it toured senior centers in the Bronx, interest in the play inspired an independent film company to make a documentary about it, entitled "Women of Hodson." The film incorporated interviews, scenes from rehearsal and performance, and audience response, and dynamically conveyed the group's sense of purpose and spirit.

Since then, two more plays were created and performed. *Holiday Heat 1979* dramatized the current oil shortage and how it affected the elderly; and *Grandma's Home Remedy Show* chronicled changing patterns of health care, from the home remedies of half a century ago to the clinic care of today. Like celebrities, people in the group spoke on radio and television on themes such as aging and health care and performed scenes from the plays. Of course, true to their origins, they also brought the plays to centers in their neighborhood.

The group had come a long way. They were excited about sharing stories, understood how to make a play, and had gained confidence and skill in performing for others. Although none of them had ever acted professionally before, they now took theater seriously. Much of what made for a successful group was their learning to deal with specific problems as they arose. Members had different levels of ability. Some could move around more easily than others. Some had problems with seeing, hearing, speaking, and remembering. They were emotionally different: some were alert, interested, curious and enthusiastic, while others tended to be withdrawn, confused, depressed or bitter. But, no matter what her physical or psychological capacity, each person was unique, important, and could make her distinct contribution. Each person was able to grow and change within the group.

Each workshop session had a similar structure. Beginning informally, each member was accounted for. There was discussion about how things were going, and who was out for a clinic appointment or illness. Members were not made to feel guilty about illness. However, they did feel it was their responsibility to inform the group, so their absence could be taken into consideration for rehearsal or performance. The importance of each individual was stressed.

The workshops formally began with physical exercises to bring the group together, increase group concentration, release tensions, and tune up the body. The goals of the physical work were to develop strength and confidence in the ability to move, to reinforce a positive self-image, to gain self-respect and physical and verbal assertiveness. The specific exercises were adapted from "aches and pains sessions" where people talked about what was bothering them. Often exercises focused on one individual's problems and taught the group about how to handle a specific problem. For example, the group learned breathing exercises for shortness of breath and high blood pressure, massages for muscle stiffness and circulation, and joint exercises for arthritis and bursitis.

After the warm-up, drama skills were developed through improvisations. These often took the form of problem-solving explorations based on the life experiences of the members. All the content we uncovered was considered confidential and kept within the group. Each work session ended with an evaluation in which members had a chance to air any problems they had with the work, with others in the group, or with the way we were doing things. Through this activity, group members learned to sum up the activities of each session and to plan the following one. They began functioning as performers and administrators, setting up informal as well as formal networks of communication, which helped resolve problems and which extended beyond the limits of group time.

On one occasion, Estelle, a proud and dignified woman, was having trouble finding her way around. At the beginning of the session, Estelle had not said hello to her friend, Mary, who noticed this with a jeweler's eye and subsequently became angry and refused to talk to Estelle. In turn, Estelle, coming from Charleston, South Carolina, claimed she knew an affront when she saw one, and proceeded to make nasty remarks about Mary. There seemed to be a misunderstanding brought on by different cultural styles. Despite appearances, it turned out not to be an encounter between Estelle's slow southern manner and Mary's tough, Harlem "cool." During the evaluation, we discovered that Estelle was worried about her eyesight; her glaucoma had worsened, and an operation might be necessary. She had not slighted Mary; she had not *seen* her. The friends embraced, and now everyone started to ask Estelle about her eyesight and to offer advice.

In another case, Sally, a small, fragile woman of eighty-three, was thought to be senile. During a performance, she became disoriented and wandered aimlessly around the stage. Some members felt she should not perform because she confused others when she lost her way. "When someone is lost," one of the women suggested, "what they need is a guide." And so the problem was solved by assigning her a buddy to help guide her through the play. Sally made good use of her buddy, calling her at home to go over her parts and to discuss other problems. She improved incredibly, seemed twenty years younger, and was able to take on leading roles in subsequent plays.

The degree of commitment to others grew within the group. This was revealed most dramatically in an incident involving Carrie, an energetic, eighty-seven-year-old who lived alone in the projects. She loved creating roles. During one session, she played a grandmother who was watching her grandchild disco dance. Carrie was moving her feet lightly to the music when suddenly she grabbed her heart. Knowing she had a heart condition, we insisted she stop. After a couple of months rest, during which Carrie was treated like a favored child, she rejoined the group, asserting that the group's concern gave her something to live for and pulled her through. Carrie informed us that, "If I'm going out, I want to go out dancing." She began to give others useful information about how they could take care of their hearts while continuing to act.

Of course, not all problems are resolved so easily. One member became ill while performing at a senior center. She claimed we were trying to poison her. Reassurances from the group that this was not the case fell on deaf ears, and she stopped coming. Subsequently, I called her and discovered that her boyfriend insisted that acting was "the work of the devil," that she would have to choose between him and the group, and she chose her boyfriend.

In the process of creating living history plays, members of Hodson Senior Center not only developed a deeper understanding of the roles they played within the group and the play but also learned to think about larger social issues and to see themselves within a broader historical context—all of which became evident when the entire theater group participated in demonstrations against the cutbacks in services to senior centers. For Evelyn Virgo, a jolly, hefty woman who always spoke her mind, it meant becoming the Center's president and acquainting herself with a wide range of issues that affected senior citizens. When two congressmen came to solicit the senior vote, it was Evelyn who stood up and proudly delivered her opening monologue from *Three Generations*, citing how during the war years they, the seniors, had helped run the city, and raised families besides. Gathering a full head of steam, Evelyn told the congressmen that the time had come to listen to the elderly and to speak to their needs. No longer sitting quietly, the members of the Center cheered Evelyn's eloquent performance on their behalf.

2. *A SCENARIO OF* THREE GENERATIONS

Act I—Prologue: Each person comes forward, introduces herself, and tells her lineage as far back as she can go: first her name and where she was born, then her parents' names and where they were born, and even back further. Each monologue ends with a comment about the performer's role in the family. Evelyn proudly proclaims, "I was the ninth of thirteen children, and it was fun down on the farm." Estelle, swaying with her hands on her hips, smiles and says, "I was the youngest and I'm a southern belle."

Act I—Scene 1: "Growing Up": Home on the farm in Claredon County, South Carolina in the 1920s. Ten children come in from school and do their daily chores. Sally cleans out the tray in the icebox before the iceman comes. Evelyn and her sisters wash the dirty clothes and hang them out to dry, while giggling about their boyfriends. Estelle and the younger children pick cotton in the field. Anne collects the eggs from the chicken coop, chasing two old lady chickens off their nest so that she can get to the eggs. Act I ends with Mama ringing the dinner bell and all the kids running home from their chores for Mama's good cooking—hot corn bread, collard greens, and ham hocks.

Act II—Prologue: "The War Years": Place—New York City in the 1940s. In the prologue each woman marches forward and tells her World War II story. Evelyn tells how she raised two children, while she and her husband worked overtime at the Jack Frost Sugar Factory. During that time the workers went out on strike; she was shop steward. Sally explains she was married, but did not have children and "that was that."

Act II—Scene 1: "The Factory": Erma tells her story while the performers set up a garment factory scene behind her, sewing uniforms for the boys overseas. Erma explains she would get up at dawn, get the kids off to school and go to work. One morning, the kids were ill and she arrived late to work. She runs onto the stage and tells the foreman that her kids are sick and the babysitter is late. When the foreman docks her pay, the other women angrily protest. This incident sets off complaints about the high prices of food, poor working conditions, and the struggle to unionize the shop. Fortunately for the foreman, the whistle blows, so the women close their sewing machines, and hurry off home to take care of their children and prepare dinner.

Act II—Scene 2: "The Food-Rationing Line": The women line up to buy their groceries with ration books. They shiver in the cold and end up getting less meat, sugar, and butter than they need. Some joke about the situation, while others impatiently wait to be served.

Act II—Scene 3: "Henrietta's Tuesday Night Open-Prayer Meeting": Onstage, friends, relatives, and neighbors gather to share information about the weather, the prices, and the war. Anna reads a letter from her husband in Pearl Harbor. Ethlin is told about her brother, missing in action. Together, everyone prays for the boys' safe return home. Then the women, in harmony, sing "He's Got the Whole World in His Hands," clapping their hands and dancing to the rhythm of the song while the audience is asked to join in. They realize it is late, time to go, and say good-bye until the next Tuesday.

Act III—Prologue: "Modern Times": The prologue opens with the women humming "We Shall Overcome," the song of the civil rights movement that ushered in modern times for the Hodson Drama Group members. Elizabeth comes forward and tells about her trip back down to her hometown, Montgomery, Alabama, in the late 1960s. When she returned there, she found that there were no more "colored" water fountains, that stores were hiring "colored folk," and that she could sit in the front of the bus with white people. After Elizabeth, each woman comes forward to talk about what had happened in her life over the last twenty years. Husbands died, children moved away, and women retired from work. Anne explains how she lives alone in the public housing project and comes to Hodson Senior Center every day. It is the center of her life.

Act III—Scene 1: "Anna Rouse's Apartment House in the Bronx": Grandma comes to see how her grandchildren are doing. Disco blares from the radio, and Mother Rouse has to shout to remind her teenage daughter to do the laundry at the laundromat. Evelyn pays little attention; she is too busy dancing with sister Sally. After carefully surveying the scene, Grandma slowly gets up and joins her grandchildren, "shaking her booty" to the music. Mother shouts at them all to stop and move on to the day's business. The children leave for school, and Grandma goes off to the senior center to "watch the boys go by."

Act III—Scene 2: "Hodson Senior Center's Monthly Birthday Party": Grandma enters and tells about her visit with her grandchildren. Everyone talks about how kids today "have no respect," "do whatever they want," "don't listen," and yet, "are loved just the same." The birthday party begins with couples gaily waltzing to the tune of the "Anniversary Waltz." After explaining what Hodson Senior Center means to them, the group sings the finale song:

> Lean on me when you're not strong
> I'll be your friend
> I'll help you carry on
> For it won't be long that

I'm going to need somebody to lean on.
Just call on me, sister
When you need a hand
I might have a problem that you'll understand.
We all need somebody to lean on.

After the show the players go into the audience and collect memories and reactions from the viewers. For all of them the show brings back echoes of a time lived and gone. They speak of having witnessed the change from kerosene lamps to electric lights, from horse and buggy to jet airplane, from Mama's home cooking to frozen T.V. dinners, and from the large, extended, rural family to the inner city nuclear family.

3. FINDING A THEATRICAL FORM

An important aspect of the living history play is that cultural values are revealed in the context of the circumstances that shaped them. In uncovering the link between their individual lives and the broader historical framework, the women in the Hodson Drama Group gained dignity, a sense of identity and belonging, and an understanding of the particularity of their lives as well as their commonality with others. From oral history and life review, the group learned to value and to create plays that conveyed the drama of *their* history—history as they experienced it. In our highly literate and technological society, there is a built-in tendency to formalize and objectify historical data, which means placing a heavy reliance on written documentation and formal histories. The tendency to objectify history goes along with the view of history as a science: as something that is readily measurable in time and place and that is analyzed and interpreted by "the experts." And so the isolated individual tends to see history taking place outside herself or himself, located somewhere in the past, a sequence of actions performed by other men and women more prominent on the world stage.

When the women began working on living history plays, they didn't understand history as a complex process of people's struggle for power, and as the ideas, myths, and rituals that shape a time and a place. What they possessed was a personal history that they could never fully understand because it still remained unconnected to the historical forces which had, in part, shaped their lives. To live not merely *of* one's time, but *in* one's time, demands cultivating a historical imagination, and means going beyond the self. Rather than view history as fixed in the past, they came to understand it as a process significantly linked to the present. Through creative dramatics, they were able to speak about their particular ethnic drama and to connect it to United States history as a whole.

In most senior citizens' centers, drama groups have adapted Broadway musicals such as *Gigi*, *My Fair Lady*, and *Around the World in Eighty Days*. Undoubtedly, doing such plays is entertaining, but they do not give a sense of purpose that living history plays provide. The women of the Hodson Drama Group discovered their own voices and acquired a confidence in their own vision of life as they learned to recognize the importance of the playwright's choice of themes. The overwhelmingly enthusiastic response of the audience reflected the deep identification of the audience with the performers. Both gained respect for their lives and a shared understanding of their role in history. They saw again the struggles they had dealt with and reviewed their lives with new compassion and objectivity.

In transforming life review into theater, there are essentially six steps:

1. Learning the appropriate theater skills
2. Selecting a theme
3. Collecting stories and other cultural and historical information
4. Selecting the historical material
5. Developing the scenario, rehearsing, and setting the play
6. Performance

1. For many older adults who have never considered acting, a traditional theater class is threatening. In working on *Three Generations*, theatrical skills and life experience were integrated whenever possible. For the first year, Hodson Drama Group learned theater games and improvisational skills. Exercises fostered trust and associative responses. Each session contained a physical warm-up to prepare the actor's tool, the body. Voice work included yoga breathing exercises, singing, and musical "jamming." In a group sound jam, for example, people listen and fit their own voice into a musical picture created by the group. Different forms of this exercise include simply singing a chord, jamming to a melody, playing with rhythms, and "sound and motion." When the group jammed

on songs from World War II, it was fascinating to discover that Anne remembered "Don't Take My Darling Boy Away" about "the people who declare the wars and the mothers who have no say," a song with a point of view about World War II that I had not heard. When they recalled songs from childhood, one song led to the next. They collected mama's lullabies, fever songs, and southern game songs.

When we came to do character work, emphasis was first placed on physicalization, which essentially involved remembering how grandmother walked, talked, and gestured. Exercises for heightened body sensitivity, initially done to develop an awareness of body parts, later were coupled with word or sound associations.

Members reenacted the physical characteristics of each age: childhood, adolescence, young adulthood, middle age, and old age. They chose people from their lives whom they enacted in the group: their children, relatives, acquaintances, workers, friends, and neighbors. Mary recalled her mother cooking in the kitchen and replayed the scene in *Three Generations*, sharing her mother's special recipes for ham hocks and apple pie.

While collecting stories, the group proceeded from character work to role playing. One way of doing this was using gibberish to convey tonality of expression. The conviction is that it is not only what you say but how you say it that tells the story. In one exercise, people came to understand the different ways of saying yes. They said yes in ways that meant yes, no, maybe: they said yes to express love, hate, anger, boredom. Soon they became sensitive to the nuances of expression and had a wonderful time as well. Carrie discovered her sister usually said yes to mean *not now*, and played out a childhood scene in which she was her reticent younger sister. She relived and reintegrated her feeling about her sister through this discovery.

2. Time was set aside for discussion of themes for plays. After about two months, the group chose a theme to concentrate on. Having already created *A Slice of Our Lives*, the group wanted to deepen its understanding of the specific experience that women had. The men had already dropped out, so the discussion became more intimate. We decided to explore the changing role of women in the family. All the women agreed that family life as they knew it was in trouble since the mass migration of black people to the north. The large extended family had broken down. Most of the older women

had no family around them. They found it hard to adapt to new ways of getting day-to-day support. Clearly the drama group helped people. *Three Generations* was about a central and shared problem—the dissolution of the close-knit extended family, which left them lonely and with little connection to their past lives.

3. Collecting information took a couple of months. The group rediscovered the routines of daily living during each decade of their lives by recalling stories, songs, dances, and fashions. Some specific techniques for eliciting memories came from photographs, interviews, letters, newspaper articles, and personal props and costumes.

Interviewing was an important technique for getting material for scenes. The aim was primarily to elicit information and to explore. The interviewer functioned like a medium whose own presence, interests, and questions conjured corresponding memories; these provided insight into how people thought about events and what they perceived their own role to have been. Different structures for interviewing developed out of the needs of the work-in-progress. In a one-to-one interview, for example, the grandmother questioned her daughter about the whereabouts of her grandchildren in order to gather information about family life in "Modern Times." In another improvisation, the group interviewed a single character. The union members played by the group interviewed the boss about his company and job requirements for women during World War II.

After the interviewing was done, the group discussed what was said and what was not said to discover what was acceptable and what was taboo. Each interviewee had a chance to reflect on the material that came up: what felt important, unexpected, true, distorted. Other members responded with their own recollections. At first the women claimed they had no opinion and were uninformed about history. Then people spoke of their work experience. We discovered that several members of the group had participated in labor conflicts during the war. Evelyn, who played the foreman in the factory scene, had been a shop steward and participated in a strike. Other women had supported the no-strike pledge taken by nearly all recognized unions during the war. People discovered their connection to history.

4. Once scenes were collected from everyone's life, the most difficult and important decision-making process began. Of the many

social, political, and cultural forces that underlay the individual life stories, we had to select which larger themes to illuminate. During this time, members began to see themselves as part of the fabric of history, not outside it. They saw how race and sex prejudice had affected them. They better understood their real choices in life and often reintegrated painful experiences in a new context. Thus in *Three Generations*, the farm scene was selected because it showed the fun and hardships of living in a large, extended family in which everyone felt needed and had responsibilities. Also, in "The War Years" section of the play, they decided to have a factory scene rather than one set in the home, since nearly all the women had entered the factory work force at that time.

While creating an opening to "Modern Times," we spoke about which historical events signified the biggest change in how they viewed themselves. For the Blacks, it was the civil rights movement, whereas for the Jews, it was the Holocaust. Since this was primarily a Black group, they selected the civil rights movement. Family scenes set in the living room focused on cultural and political conflicts. The improvisations between grandparents, parents, and children dramatized arguments about dashikis and corn braids, about freedom marches, and radical black power groups. The group recalled the gospel song, "We Shall Overcome," and sang it together holding hand over hand. This song linked the older and younger generation in the sixties. In the play, the group hummed the song, as Estelle told of her home visit to Alabama and of her astonishment at all the changes she witnessed.

5. Once scenes had been determined, committees were set up for developing the play, rehearsing the scenes, and getting the props and costumes together. Such a procedure helped the group acquire a conscious sense of its creative and critical powers. In each committee, every person found a character to develop in her own particular way. A committee acted out an improvised scene for other drama group members. People watched and listened carefully because after the scene was over, individuals would volunteer to re-enact what they saw, trying to capture the essential dynamics of the scene. We called this process "instant replay" since it was like watching a sports playback on television. After the replay, when the actors in the committee had a chance to see themselves, they would then play the scene again. This back-and-forth process helped them clarify the plot, and set the lines and characterizations in their

scenes. While repeating this scene, each actor had the artistic liberty of adding her own touches. In this way, all the characters and their conflicts became clearer to everyone in the group. They had all participated in developing every scene.

Our working principle was that if you know *who* you are, *where* you are, and *what* the problem is, you never have to worry because you are always able to find your own words to express the story.

This approach to collective play creation was particularly well suited for working with senior citizens. At Hodson it was not uncommon for someone to be out sick or at a doctor's appointment during rehearsal. Using this method of story setting, the entire group took responsibility for understanding the scenes. Through instant replay, "understudies" were always available. Before performance, we would find out who was absent, assign parts, and simply talk through the scenes. At first this was a scary and unsettling way to work, but after a while, it lent its own brand of excitement to performing. Each performance was unique and held surprises for everyone.

Eventually, through continued performance, the play settled into a stable form. Unfortunately a script of *Three Generations* was never made. This play came and went in the tradition that brought it about—the passing down of stories from generation to generation.

6. Performances were always extraordinary events for the drama group as well as the audience. Each performance began with a warm-up that included the audience. Actors and audience shook their arms above their heads, rotated their shoulders, swung their legs, stretched their bodies, and let their voices sing out in call and response, so that the tale could be told. We had structured this like a celebration, a ritual preparation that was shared by all.

Always, after the performance, the audience was encouraged to share their recollections with the drama group. After one performance, my mother, herself a grandmother, came up to me. She dried her teary eyes, as she explained that I might now be better able to understand how hard it had been for her to raise my brother and me during World War II. She poured out stories from the war years that I probably would never have heard if it had not been for *Three Generations.*

During one performance, Irma and Ethlin were greeted with a standing ovation when they traced their lineage back to Panama. As a result of the play, a number of Panamanian immigrants found each

other, and a Bronx-Panama group was formed. After another performance, members of the Center reenacted their own version of
Three Generations in an exuberant exchange of life experiences.

At the Center of the Story

Grace Worth

> There are stories within stories. Let us ask about them, begin-
> ning with the stories where time counts most and ending with
> those where it counts least, going from time to timelessness,
> from time to lifetime to moment.[1]—John S. Dunne

A sunny April afternoon, 1980. The gathering group of twelve
older persons moved slowly into the large second-floor room of the
Over-the-Rhine Senior Center in Cincinnati. Since September,
many of them had been coming twice weekly to a city-wide program
for older people sponsored by the Arts and Humanities Resource
Center (AHRC).[2] Today there were far fewer than the usual sixty or
more. The topic of this particular segment, Personal History/
Creative Writing, must have been intimidating to many of those unfamiliar with writing skills beyond their elementary school experience.

I asked everyone to help arrange the long tables in an L-shape so
we could be close together. After Sister Joan Leonard, the director
of AHRC, introduced me, there was that familiar waiting-silence of
all first classes when my thoughts run a thousand miles a second,
and my words come slow and stumbling. The tape recorder in the
background caught our beginning.

I told them briefly how this twelve-week class was related to what
had gone before:

> During the time you have been coming to the other sessions of
> this project, you have heard the story of the growth of music in
> Cincinnati, the history of dance, of art, of the theatre. You
> have been looking at many things which were taking place in
> the growth of the city. Now, in this class we will move to the
> story of the people—you—the story of you in relationship to
> your home place, your people, the events of your life. And we
> will catch some of those stories and put them in writing.

Before we begin, I'm wondering, have any of you done any writing before? *Any* kind of writing at all?

A murmur of no's, and then Mattie said yes, she did some writing. I nodded for her to go on, and she said she wrote cards, Christmas cards, and cards for birthdays. I nodded again, and she continued, "You know, I writes my name at the bottom of the card. And I writes the envelope too and puts my address in the corner." The others were all listening seriously, and the fact came forcefully home to me: most of these people considered it an accomplishment to do the most rudimentary form of "writing." They replied no to my questions about writing letters, or grocery lists or lists of any kind. Mattie pointed to her head and said, "I writes it all up here!"

I then told them why I was here:

> I like to write and I like to teach others to write; mostly, I love *words*. The wonderful sounds of them—like the way you just said that, Mattie—and the variety of ways we can use them. I like the way our language reveals not only what we want to tell about, but our inside selves. You know how we are caught by the way a child sometimes says something in his own special way? And we want to remember to tell others? Or how we cherish a particular expression of our mother or father? We each have special ways of speaking. We're just not always aware of the beauty of our own personal way with words.

> The turn of a phrase, the words, the rhythms of a story told. In the other sessions you have played with clay and made pots, you have moved your bodies in different ways, making dance, you have played around with melodies to make song. So, over the next few weeks we will play with words to tell the stories of our lives; we will play around until we find the right words to tell not only the outward happenings of those stories, but the inside meanings, too.

Someone questions, "Will we learn to use good English?"

> It depends on what you mean by "good." To be honest, we won't be spending much time on what you might have studied in school called "good English grammar." We'll learn when *not* to use it, and mostly how to hear our *own* good English, and when to use *that*. We'll be paying a lot of attention to your

own way of speaking in order to discover its special beauty and power, and we'll be working to learn how to use your own language creatively.

They seem interested and curious about what I might mean by all this.

There are two things I want to tell you, and then I'll stop talking and you can begin your part. Whenever I sit down to write, and whenever I work with people in writing classes, one fact keeps impressing itself on me. It is this:

We seem always to know more than we can tell. I write this on the board, and pause. They begin to nod their heads and to smile knowingly to each other.

And this fact sits side-by-side in me with another which I can best tell you through a story about my nephew Jason. When Jason was four years old, my sister Pat, who had not seen him for some time, arrived for a visit. Looking down at him, she said, "Jason! You've gotten so big!" He looked up at her and answered, "But Aunt Pat, you know what?" "No, what?" "I'm really even bigger than this!"

I write this last on the board with the other. Again there is a knowing nodding of heads and quiet comments of yes, that's so, isn't that something.

What Jason was telling is what we all feel at times. It is what we often try to recover as we tell the different stories of our lives, striving in the very telling to find the significance. Telling the stories reminds us that we do know more than we can tell; and in the telling we come sometimes into something bigger than we knew, and we are part of *that*. This is what we will be doing together here. So, before our time is gone, let's begin.

And a little fear comes over me, a kind of awe before the human persons here, and all they hold un-told, an awe at putting myself in the position of being able to unlock closed doors and open old trunks. Then, another fear that *nothing* might happen. They have an understanding of what I have been saying, yet most of them are afraid or at least hesitant before the pencil and paper in front of them. My goals are two-fold: first, that they come to a more conscious appreciation of their own language; and second, that they experience within themselves the process involved in the craft of the written word. I look around the semi-circle and ask them what they are about to ask me: "How shall we begin?"

Each person had a piece of yellow lined tablet paper and a pencil in front of him or her. I told them to begin by putting a small square in the middle of the paper and to mark it with an "x." The square represented the home they lived in when they were about ten years old. The boundaries of the paper were the approximate boundaries of their home "territory," one edge being perhaps the big street over there that you weren't allowed to cross, or the creek you never walked beyond; another edge, the cemetery down the road a bit, or the street with the corner grocery store where you bought milk and bread. For about five minutes, each one was to fill in within those boundaries a kind of map of the home-place, noting as many details as could be recalled—street or road names, names of neighbors and friends, stores, churches—not in the way a professional map-maker would do it, but in a personal way, indicating anything which had special meaning such as a big rock by the creek, a willow tree, an abandoned wagon. Finally, I said, this was not an art contest: they should make notes and markings on their maps in whatever fashion suited them. They picked up the pencils and began.

A serious quiet came over the room. I moved among them, helping those who looked at a loss. Mr. Bradley didn't want to do it. I said that was all right, he could just look at the paper and bring back the memories. He said it was too long ago, he didn't have anything to remember. I asked if he would listen once the others began telling their stories. He said, yes, he would like to listen. I said we needed people to listen and I hoped he would keep coming. He came almost every time, and during one of the last sessions picked up the pencil for the first time. Rosa, who had cataracts, tried to make a map, made one wobbly line—a creek or a road—and said she couldn't see. I suggested that she use the piece of paper as a frame for concentrating and thinking, even if she couldn't mark the places with the pencil. She said, "But I can't see." So I stayed with her for a few minutes, asking what was behind the house, what kind of trees, what was planted in the fields, where the road led to. Then I left her to think quietly on her own. The room was now hushed, they were all absorbed in their work. Mattie smiled and drew a big circle around her map. Eleanor began laughing out as she recalled something. Wilma looked over, smiled, then returned to her own work in a deeper state of concentration. Each was engrossed, and taking delight, in the memories which rushed to consciousness as they filled in one detail after another.

After five minutes of map-drawing, we paired off, each with a partner, to tell the story of the map—three minutes to talk, and three to listen. I encouraged them to tell about the events and persons they had remembered in relation to the places noted. Although Mr. Bradley wanted "just to listen," he told some of his own stories, which were brought to mind upon hearing his partner's. He had so much to tell he didn't want to stop when the time was up. The tape recorder caught it all: a hubbub of voices, sounds of excitement and delight, quiet talking, sudden laughter, exclamations of understanding, the voices moving in and out among one another.

When we all came back together, I asked a few questions about their memories. They said that they remembered sharp details about people, things, events which they hadn't thought of for forty or fifty years. During the sharing time, they had remembered even more than they had while making the map. With delight they mentioned one detail after another, as though all were distinctly present now, and not part of a distant past. From the rural South: a chinaberry tree, fig trees, cotton—lots of it, and memories of the picking; chestnuts in the woods, wine-making and hog-slaughtering. Rosa said she remembered mostly just "running, as a child, over the hills of Tennessee." From the city of Cincinnati: the iceman, the stockyards and their smell, the canal and the steamers, the outhouses and Batchie, the man who came at night to clean them. Bill summed it up, "It was a pretty good life, really, a working-class neighborhood with a cat-woman, a wash-woman, and all."

I told them about Joseph Campbell's book, *The Hero With a Thousand Faces*, and how he shows that all our stories are parts of one big story which tells of the life-journey of the hero. We then related this idea to their stories: What kinds of places did they have on the map? A Forbidden Place, a Secret Place, a Mysterious Place, Meeting Places and Places-to-Be-Alone. And the People? Did they have a Mean Old Witch there? A good Fairy Godmother? Father, Brother, Mother and Sister. The Good Friend. The Wise Old Uncle. The Leader. And times of Celebration, of Mourning? Of Birth and Death, of Home-Coming and of Farewells. Neither the room nor the hour could hold all the stories they had to tell. We had, I said, been doing what some would call a little myth-making with our own lives. We would be doing more of the same during the following weeks: spending some time remembering, and then some time sharing. "Some of what you remember will get told, some will go untold, but you will be telling your stories to yourselves in the remembering. And we will write some of them down." I turned to what was written on the board:

> We always know more than we can tell.
> I'm really even bigger than this.

I didn't say anything. Just smiled, and they smiled back.

I find the map-making exercise, or some form of it, essential to the process of learning creative writing because it gives the apprentice immediate access to the materials of his or her own life. It arouses, through a brief and intense process, those concrete archetypal images which contain and carry our larger story, and through which it can best be told. Carl Jung speaks about this in an essay on the relationship between psychology and poetry:

> The impact of an archetype, whether it takes the form of immediate experience or is expressed through the spoken word, stirs us because it summons up a voice that is stronger than our own. Whoever speaks in primordial images speaks with a thousand voices; he enthralls and overpowers, while at the same time he lifts the idea he is seeking to express out of the occasional and the transitory into the realm of the everenduring. He transmutes our personal destiny into the destiny of mankind, and evokes in us all those beneficent forces that ever and anon have enabled humanity to find a refuge from every peril and to outlive the longest night.
>
> That is the secret of great art, and of its effect upon us. The creative process, so far as we are able to follow it at all, consists in the unconscious activation of an archetypal image, and in elaborating and shaping this image into the finished work. By giving it shape, the artist translates it into the language of the present, and so makes it possible for us to find our way back to the deepest springs of life.

Jung's words may seem idealistic and intellectual, far removed from the people gathered together at the Over-the-Rhine Center. They do, however, accurately describe what we experienced in our writing sessions there.

During our twelve-week project, the topic and boundaries of each memory-raising activity were constructed in such a way that, without restricting the learner to too narrow a form, they served to satisfy what Wallace Stevens calls that "Blessed rage for order" of the human imagination, that human urge to give a new and personal form to the otherwise random, formless, often chaotic or painful circumstances of our lives. I adapted the basic idea of the map-making described above for a variety of memory-raising experiences. The boundaries of the map enclosed a larger world or a smaller one, the inside or the outside. During one session, for example, they made a floor plan of the inside of a childhood home, noting details such as furniture, wallpaper, floor coverings. After the one-on-one sharing, they walked in memory through the kitchen of the house and then narrowed the focus even further to items on the walls of the kitchen. They recalled calendars, religious pictures, pots and pans and cooking utensils, the clothesline strung behind the pot-bellied stove to dry the long winter underwear. And sweet potatoes roasting in the ashes in the grate; the warming oven of the wood cook stove, the ash pan and the wood box. These last two things brought back the child's work: emptying the ashes (onto the path to the chicken house), and carrying the wood in every evening before dark, every morning before school. Some few had had the luxury of a stove in the bedroom; all had memories of themselves as children getting good and warm by the stove, then running to get into bed.

They were tapping their own resources for the artistic shaping of stories, and the images flowed out: a china pattern, a special chair or table, a ceramic milk pitcher, the shape of a person's shoes, the smell and taste of a particular food. They were gathering materials and telling stories, and in the process becoming more and more aware of the emotional content which could be expressed through these small details. Listening was as vital as talking. During the sharing time, they were amazed time and again at the universality of those particulars which before had seemed important only to their individual lives and persons.

While they were getting excited over their memories, my assistant, Kate McGann, and I paid attention to the language in which they told of them. Kate began jotting down poetic phrases, particular turns of speech which struck her. I would read these back to them, pointing out their natural abilities in using language and in the art of storytelling. I now think it would have been helpful had they seen some of these examples in print during the very first sessions. Gradually they became more conscious of the unique beauty of their own words and the richness of their own way of speaking, and subsequently of the language skills associated with writing. From Kate's jottings, my memory, and the tape recorder, I found examples of—

Good beginnings:

> "Grandma was like a flower. . ."

> "Sometime ago I was driving about a mile from the house that was my birthplace. . ."

> "My father liked to sing. No notes like do, re, mi. My father liked singin' songs."

And good endings:

> "I filled with joy when I could see the yellow glow of the light in the window."

> "Gotta go bed, sis. Gotta go bed, sis."

Rhythmic repetitions:

> "Here she come again, with those grits. . .
> Come noontime, here she come again. . .
> Then come dinner, here she come again with those same grits, fixed up different again."

> "I been walkin' ever since,
> I be 86 years old,
> I been walkin' ever since."

Bits of wisdom held in simple descriptions:

> "An old iron will flatten out anything, whether it be hot or cold."

> "Tin-top roofs, you sleep so good, when it rains."

> "Sometimes we hear so differently from what people are speaking. We just have to find out what's happening."

And through it all, a natural sense of symbol and image.

Another variation of the map which I used was a kind of "guided reverie." The thoughts take on more of a dream-like quality than in the map-work, without specific anchors in space and time, and with a freer flow of meaningful images and associations. I introduced this activity during the fourth session with a reverie centered on a family dinner:

> We might call this a kind of day-dreaming. To get into the dreaming, you'll need to be comfortable and relaxed. My words will guide you through the dream, setting the scene and event, leaving time for you to fill in the particulars, just as you did on your maps.
>
> Close your eyes so you will not be distracted by the people and things or by the light in this room. Try to follow me as closely as you can, but don't worry if you start to drift off. Some of you may even want to go to sleep!
>
> Close your eyes (pause), breathe deeply (pause), relax. For awhile, empty out all your concerns and worries. Go into your inside world and leave the cares of the outside behind. Breathe slowly (pause), and deeply. (Pause.)

I continued talking, slowly and clearly, but not dramatically.

> You are sitting alone in the middle of a large room. (Pause.)
>
> You are waiting for the family dinner. (Pause.)
>
> All the others will be coming soon, so you get up and begin preparing the table before the others arrive.
>
> You set a place for everyone-how many do you need? (Pause.) Dishes (pause), eating utensils (pause), something to drink from. (Pause.)
>
> Put on everything you want-a centerpiece of some sort (pause), something to drink? (Long pause.)
>
> When the food is ready, you bring it on. (Pause.) All of the serving dishes full, and smelling so good. (Pause.) Are there rolls or bread? Don't forget butter? Bring whatever you need. (Long pause.)
>
> When the table is ready, your family begins to arrive, one by

one. You say hello to each one as they come in the door and take their places. (Long pause.) You look at them, hold hands or give a hug, saying hello and welcome. (Long pause.)

After everyone is seated, the dinner begins (pause), the food is passed (pause); there is much laughing and talking together. (Pause.)

You look around at these people, big and small, who belong to you in a special way. (Pause.) You may want to talk to certain ones. (Long pause.)

You pause from eating and take a moment to look at the things you remember-the light, the things on the walls, the furniture, whatever. (Pause.)

When the meal is finished, it is time to say good-bye. You wait by the door and say farewell to each as they all leave. (Long pause.)

And when they have all gone (pause), you sit down again, in the middle of the room alone. (Pause.) Breathe a deep good-bye (pause), and when you are ready, open your eyes and come back here.

This kind of guided reverie is apt to recall a traumatic or intense experience that arouses very strong emotions or new insights not seen before. Therefore, I usually gave them time to talk first in the large group before sharing one-on-one. It was a very quiet sharing compared to that which followed the map activities. Some were wiping away brief tears. I set a slower pace, giving enough time for them to absorb the experience, so that people might not speak up too fast, or share what they weren't quite ready to. I suggested a few minutes of quiet, a time in which they could simply reflect on the details of the dreaming, or jot down things on the paper before them. Mattie drew a diagram of the table and the places and names of those who had been there, and then wrote on the lower half of the paper, "Now no one but me." Other reveries might be constructed around a holiday celebration, moving day, spring cleaning, a birth-day, a conversation with a loved one (past or present).

When, at the beginning of the third class, I announced that we would write poems, they froze, saying they couldn't write *poetry*. "You've been writing poems all along," I said, "Just not consciously.'' To begin to look at how poetry is different from story-telling, I read a poem by William Carlos Williams. I first explained that he was a doctor who had lived in New Jersey, and that he had often written his poems between patients, because he would hear poems as people talked. The one I read is titled, ''Short Poem'':

> You slapped my face
> oh but so gently
> I smiled
> at the caress

There was an audible ''Ahhhh'' when I finished, and Grace turned to her good friend and ran her hand gently down the side of her face. A delightful discussion followed, about how few details the poem gives, and yet how vividly we felt the experience; how we could not know from the poem who the two people were, whether two women, mother and child, child and grandparent, husband and wife. But it did not matter. We had enough to know what it was about, and each of us from our own experience could say, as they had after the reading, ''Ah, yes, I know!'' So what makes a poem different from prose? As we talked I wrote on the board:

Center of the story

Less words

Special rhythm

''You probably think of poetry as something which rhymes?'' They nodded. ''That is only one kind of poetry, and probably not the best to try writing when you first begin.''

I then asked them to take one story they had already told, and try to tell it with fewer words. We then worked with these, focusing on only two tasks: choosing words or phrases essential to the ''heart'' of the story as the author felt it, and choosing how best to place them on the page. We did this together, one person volunteering his or her poem, with me writing on the board as the author dictated. Often, in process, the writer would ask the others what they thought. They became excited and involved in the process, saying yes to this phrase, no to that, put this here, yes, *that* says it. We had two poems on the board when it was (suddenly) time to go home.

Two years old—
　　Moving to Tishabee, Alabama.

Years later, I asked
　　My mother,

"Who was that little girl
　　Who stood up on the floor?"

And my mother said,
　　"That was your sister—she died."

They didn't let me know it.

　　　　　　　　　　by Mattie D. Mason

Seventy-one years ago.
Mother lying in a big brass bed.
So highly polished.

　　　　(My baby sister was born.)

Only six weeks later
Death took her away.

In a tiny casket
On my Mother's lap
She was taken to the cemetery.

　　　　(To come back again, some day.)

　　　　　　　　　　by Eleanor Keller

At the beginning of the next session, Ella Durrett wanted to read a
piece she had written down during the week. She wondered if this
could be a poem:

　　　　　Hush! Hush!
　　　　　Listen. Your daddy's talkin'.
　　　　　You know he's the man of the house.

　　　　　Be a good listener
　　　　　And you always will be
　　　　　　　in the know.
　　　　　　　　Forever.
　　　　　This is your power
　　　　　That's given to you.

After she read it, there was an appreciative, "Ahhhh." I was no longer afraid that they couldn't or wouldn't want to write poetry.

I read two more poems of Williams, and then no more established poets. We created poems ourselves, putting them on the board, deciding on spacing, words, revisions, everyone sharing the process or becoming engrossed in working on their own papers. They were now growing sensitive to the beauty of each other's language, often exclaiming, "I like the way you said that," noting the rhythm of a repeated phrase or a cultural idiom. Once when someone asked how to change a phrase from her Black dialect to "good English," Annie Gilmer spoke up before I could, "You mean *flat* English? For a poem, I think it sounds better your way!"

We continued to spend time memory-raising at the beginning of every session, and tried to find a better means to get things recorded, since so many of the participants were not at ease with writing. At one session we used tape recorders during the one-on-one sharing, but the stories became too formal, and they lost something special from the language they usually used. It was in listening to the tapes from this session and in reading the print-outs of them that Annie Gilmer first coined her phrase, "flat English." After one trial with taping, they said they preferred writing because they could be more attentive to shaping their work.

After three more weeks of poetry-writing, we made a list on the board of the items they were now aware of when writing:

Economy of words/Word choice

Special rhythms, both in the way words sound together and in the way the lines move across the page

Choice of an image to carry the meaning and emotion

Sense of a beginning/and ending

What to leave out

We had concentrated on the last three of these for the stories we put on tape. From this time on—more than half-way through—each one who came wrote in poem or story form, choosing whichever he or she wanted. Those who had been coming regularly since the beginning now showed a distinct understanding of the difference between the simple sharing of their stories, and the artistic shaping of them.

We had a total of eleven hour-long sessions, and during that time worked with two major handicaps. For one, attendance at the sessions was open, that is, anyone could drop in for any session, whether or not he had been there before. Obviously this presented a major problem in the attempt to develop continuity in our work. Sometimes there were as few as five people present, at others, as many as sixteen. However, this flexibility was an important factor for the people involved, because of transportation difficulties, illness, and other personal concerns. Some of the most enthusiastic writers were there only for the last few sessions. I had to adapt myself and the class structure to the situation, and I gave up my original expectations of a quantity of "finished" writings. We needed more time for that. Secondly, once they began shaping poems and stories, it was difficult to find the best way for those unfamiliar with paper and pencil to record theirs. The tape recorder could capture the reminiscences, but was not the best medium to use for the poems or consciously crafted stories. There were indications that, given more time, this problem also would have worked itself out. Most of the participants had hesitated to use their pencils at all during the first few sessions, Kate McGann stopped me as I was leaving the tenth session, and said excitedly, "Did you see? They couldn't wait to pick up their pencils and begin working! They wanted you and everyone else to be quiet so they could *write*!" It was true. And they were no longer wondering how to go about writing. They were absorbed in their own creative work, asking themselves, "How shall I say it? What shall I begin with? Which word here? There?"

And by the end, they had gathered, told, and heard a lot of stories. They wanted more and were sad at our ending. "You bring out so much from us," June said. "Our stories are here, but you help bring them out. That's what we need." Their coming together to write had opened the door to some ancient drive in each one to tell the stories, then in the telling to give a special shape or frame, and by the frame to proclaim a significance. Kate jotted down their good-byes: Thank you . . . I'm not makin' rhymin' poems. . . This is something I use to do—I just write about it. . . I love this . . . Thank you . . . Thank you for letting me come . . . Do we get a diploma?

Tapping the Legacy

Jeffrey Cyphers Wright

I

The planning meeting for my workshop at Countee Cullen Library took place one spring morning in 1979. Adjacent to the new Schomburg Center for Research in Black Culture, the Countee Cullen Library constitutes the primary black literary archive in New York City, if not the country. Consequently, as I expected, many of the workshop participants turned out to be very literate. In the planning session, deciding what room I should use and who would give us paper and who else would pay for xeroxing manuscripts and how long the program should last, I wondered what I could possibly teach these people of a different culture, race, and generation. The educational range in the workshop was an extra complication I hadn't begun to consider. These concerns preoccupied me as different people spoke and I faithfully wrote notes on a yellow pad. However, I did not express my qualms because I realized no one would tell me beforehand how to provide common ground or what would be important to members of the group. Only experience in the situation would satisfactorily inform me of these things. Almost as if in response to my secret doubts and fears, the library people maintained an air of assurance, like a roomful of books. From our vantage point behind massive old oak tables we could see out the back window ailanthus trees, also known as "the tree of heaven."

Perhaps it was in anticipation of future accomplishments, or the gentility of drinking rich coffee in china under a bust of Paul Laurence Dunbar, or maybe it was just some minor scheduling conflict that prompted me to volunteer to teach two workshops on Wednesdays instead of one! We decided the workshop would get a hundred dollars from the library to pay for typing and other expenses. Teachers & Writers promised to publish the writings produced in the workshop.[1]

The library was sort of enchanting. Plants thrived languorously on every available sill. A gray-headed woman offered me a coleus. High above the books great murals by Aaron Douglas traced the development of black people in North America. Banjo and saxophone music was depicted by concentric spirals, the sound waves reaching a preacher and washing over hoeing women. An old man attended by children was opening a book furtively to the candle of knowledge which flickered in the oppressive night. These paintings were illustrations to *God's Trombones*, James Weldon Johnson's cycle of seven poems based on the major themes of great gospel preachers.

God's Trombones afforded a bridge from literature to religion, and, via the murals, to art. That blend of literature, art, and religion was likely, through its diversity, to appeal to a variety of interests, making such material a natural opener. A young man working with the library knew the first poem by heart—the poem which recreates a sermon on the Creation. When he powerfully recited it at our first workshop, the feeling of grace left in its wake made our age and racial differences diminish, and apprehension was replaced with curiosity about our mutual Protestant and rural backgrounds.

II

In a workshop conducted in a library, as opposed to one in a senior center, recruitment of members becomes a big part of the job. In that effort, one of the librarians escorted me around the neighborhood to churches and community centers where we met and talked with prospects. We also passed out five hundred flyers which described the workshop and invited all to come. These efforts to get the word out were rewarded: about fifteen people came down to the cool and secluded basement auditorium the first morning we met. They came for different reasons. Some came because an interested friend dragged them along. Others were just plain curious, and a few came to write that novel they had always felt they had in them.

They were stately, these kings and queens and grandmas and seniors of Harlem, dressed in velvet suits with matching hats, wearing simulated pearls and gold bangles. They had stories to tell whether they knew it or not, and I wanted to hear them. My first step in becoming acquainted was to share some appropriate details of my own background and to encourage reciprocity on their part.

As we first got to know each other a little over cookies and juice, I admitted I had never taught a workshop before, but assured them I had attended some excellent ones, some doozies. I said I had some good ideas and asked them at this point what their expectations were and, specifically, what kinds of writing each of them was interested in. This is a delicate time in a workshop; you have to give and take the right amounts. As I asked for their suggestions, I sensed an undertone which accused me of ignorance: "I thought *you* were the teacher"; it was a kind of defensiveness, an expectation that I would guide them. Yet in order to guide them I had to address their needs and aims, so I said it was my design to codirect, rather than direct. I said I needed to know something about each of them and what they wanted to do. I explained carefully that I knew a lot about writing and could provide models and assignments, but that I was also anxious to help them do whatever kinds of writing they wanted to pursue.

The variety of responses, ranging from an interest in autobiography and community history to polite reserve, indicated the difficulty of appeasing everyone and ultimately led me to develop the "double assignment" assignment, which I will explain later.

In preparing for that first workshop, I selected a poem that conveyed a concrete idea, that would be easy to grasp, and that would serve as an easily applicable model. "Mother to Son," by Langston Hughes, gave them a model of a "direct address poem." Practically all the people were mothers and grandmothers, so they identified immediately with the "I" of the poem and her sentiment. As one of the members read the poem to the group, I was delighted and encouraged when several of the members expressed familiarity with it. Incidentally, those who were already acquainted with the poem came to form the nucleus of the group.

The workshop soon acquired a flexible agenda that began with everyone reading his or her work based on the previous week's model. The others in turn would respond. I encouraged personal comments rather than literary criticism. After everyone had read his or her piece, I would pass out xeroxed copies of the model for next week's assignment, and we would all study and discuss it. There were only two "rules": everyone must write and no one should interrupt anyone else. Neither rule was hard and fast.

It wasn't long before the topic of race surfaced. I appreciated the novelty of the situation. The people realized that my ignorance of their culture wasn't manifested in repugnance, but rather curiosity. They sensed my respect for them, their age, and abundance of experience. They opened up accordingly as the weeks went by and shared vast chunks of their lives. It became easy for me to feel secure with the directions they took as it became clear just how much more experience they had than I did. But sometimes I had to assert myself; to defend someone's writing, for instance, if it fell under attack by one of the other members.

In working with the elderly, the question of leadership requires special consideration. The young are accustomed to being deferent in respect to people older than themselves. But in the writing workshop the traditional roles were reversed. In general, I ran the show; but this tradition of deference served as a cushion when any disputes arose and offered a nice precedent for me to accept alternatives if I was confused or confusing, or if they simply weren't interested in one of my writing ideas or models.

III

All those who stuck it out long enough to leave a sense of friendship with me were delightful in different ways. Harmonizing their various qualities was not always as easy as appreciating them. One woman whose charm reigned over us in a humble, undemanding way was Mamie Walker.

Often Mamie would be there half an hour early to arrange the chairs. She rode the train all the way down from Pelham Bay in the Bronx. Mamie was the most diminutive, and seemingly the eldest; her quiet attentiveness exerted an influence on the group. She never, for example, spoke ill of anything (except love), or spoke out of turn, prompting me to think of the generalization, "old people are wise." Indeed, to me she was an envoy of the elves.

Mamie really enjoyed writing scenes and scenarios from her life. When she told about growing up in Jefferson County, Georgia, she had a way of introducing the right details so they involved the reader in her blend of whimsy and calculation. Of her teenage first impressions in her family's new home, Charleston, South Carolina, she wrote: "King Street was a main shopping center. The lights were clear bulbs, eleven in a row, hanging across the street from left to right. I tried to count every lightbulb." Mamie's eyes grinned contagiously, but a mysterious impenetrability declared her respect for the hardships of life:

A Slave to Humanity

"Work is love made visible."—Kahlil Gibhran

You know you could buy material for 10¢ a yard.
They used to have a Silver's 5 & 10
& you could buy nice material
& you know how girls are—they like
to have a lot of dresses,
they say, "Such & such has more dresses than me."
So I would take their money
& buy the material & make their dresses.

Mamie never missed a meeting or an assignment.

One of the women who dropped out of the group early wrote a large piece called "R-Day." The big R stood for Religion. Katherine, a somewhat reticent person, was rightfully proud of her work and shared it with us. She described the preparation and celebration that marked "R-Day": "Sunday we would always have dessert. Also ice-tea." The nods and mumbles of recognition as Katherine read her piece made me feel I'd hit a deep vein. This was what I was aiming for: the details and familiars that were common and dear in large part to a whole culture. I wanted to draw out in particular those kinds of recognizable things. Responding to Katherine's details, for example, Mamie affirmed that a pink bow was *de rigueur* for little girls. In this case, however, my zeal mixed with my inexperience to trip me on a point of ignorance.

I suggested that Katherine, in her piece, list the sacraments rather than simply write "on the table lay the blessed sacraments." The truth was I didn't know what the sacraments were. And there I was, the only person in the room who didn't know what they were, and ironically the very person directing them toward these mutually recognizable familiar things.

Katherine reacted to my well-meaning but meddlesome directions with affronted silence. One of the members seemed to understand my awkward position and mediated, counseling a compromise. She also said something like, "We're here to learn, and Jeffrey's the teacher." She said this a little reluctantly, and Katherine even more reluctantly changed the wording. By this time I was telling her not to, but the damage had been done. I think this incident contributed largely to Katherine's premature departure from our group.

It is discouraging to everyone when members drop out. As leader

I thought about what I might have done to precipitate Katherine's decision not to come. One must be careful to include everyone, to favor no one. Singling out aspects of someone's writing must be done in a reinforcing way. Some people, such as Katherine, can fade into the background, and these quiet people must be drawn out of themselves and into the group. I think that the common elements of class assignments promote a sense of community. An invaluable gesture is directly soliciting the less verbal members' comments and appraisals of the "community" of work that's being presented. A disruptive component in a workshop, such as someone who talks incessantly, must be dealt with firmly for the sake of the group.

Elizabeth Booker was the woman who taught me how to deal with a nonstop talker. Elizabeth did not react well to my efforts to contain her, and she also dropped out of the group early on. I found this raconteuse delightful but realized that letting her monopolize the conversation was deadly to the group. She had a way of blending stories in a seamless fashion so that they never ended! The stories were actually unbelievable, and I think the others were slightly embarrassed at her spontaneous candor. I must say, though, it was Elizabeth's impromptu accounts, and my trying to deal with them, that first sparked me to transcribe a poem from someone's talk.

My Friend

I had a little fish
    with only one eye.
Something was wrong
    with the other one.
    I loved him
    & he loved me.

But a black fish hurt
my poor little goldfish.
So I put some green stuff
    in there
    & now he's OK.
I'm trying to train him.

Although Elizabeth could have talked forever, she never wrote one line. Her reveries generally lacked such beginnings and ends as this poem has. When she spoke, the other members would begin to sigh and look at the floor or ceiling, seemingly beseeching me to do something to stop her. Of course, it was up to me to do something, but this was my first go 'round, and I was more prepared to discuss James Baldwin or Nikki Giovanni than to deal with practical affairs. Precisely because there was generally no "beginning" or "end," I soon realized I would have to appear suddenly enlightened and call on someone else with a specific question like, "What was *your* first Halloween costume, Mamie?" In an effort to bring Elizabeth into the group and include the others simultaneously, I asked them to suggest topics for her to write about. Their offerings were juicy: ghost stories, runaway tales, a list of "personal firsts." This was all fine except that Elizabeth was raring to *talk* about each of these subjects immediately upon their mention. At one point, I asked her to write a description or portrait of Violet Walker, one of the members. Since the two were strangers, Elizabeth had to take time out from talking to observe Violet.

Violet was generous and easygoing. Often she was the first to exclaim admiration for a fellow member's writing. Her proper English speech resembled the way she carried herself. Her manner was assertive, but balanced by a quick sense of humor. The formal exuberance of her writing was a mixture of her tropical Jamaican background and the traditional English education she received there. For her, I discovered Claude McKay; we both enjoyed our mutual learning adventure, reading his autobiography that began in rural Jamaica and ended with soirees in New York.

Violet would always include in her work whatever I had indicated was missing at the previous session. I found the method of "preview" criticism better than revision at this early stage in my workshop career. Violet's poems became jam-packed with color and aroma, flora and fauna. She really wanted to depict a childhood gone not only for her, but for everyone. In addition she was adept at writing Shakespearean sonnets, to which she had been introduced as a child.

For Violet, as for so many of the elderly, the church and its scriptures have been momentous both in ordering her social life and providing it with depth and focus. This was evinced in many of the group's writings by the sort of ease with which they referred to good, evil, love, hate, and sorrow. The songs, the ritual, the compassion and well-being, the starched and ironed and spotless cotton of the church were constant loci in Violet's work. Imagine what a fine feeling Violet J. Campbell sustains early on a Sunday as she walks to church, her mind confirmed in its direction and in the anticipation of enjoying her fellow adherents.

A Dream

I dreamt of a mountain high and steep.
There I was toiling up towards the top.
Then near the top I was stunned by fear.
Out of nowhere a man appeared,
with extended arms
He helped me up to the top.
That hand to me was that of God, because of its
gentle and kindly touch.
Then and there I vowed to serve Him more.
Looking around I saw a crowd.
In that crowd was my mother who has long
gone on before, beckoning me to follow her.
We crossed a rippling stream to a great green panorama.
Then she disappeared from view leaving me alone.
A "beautiful garden" of assorted flowers I saw there.
What an array of colors!
It seemed so real and inviting
while other dreams I had before were so frightening.

Another one of the more regular attenders was Aida Richardson, who met with us until she went to Alaska for a vacation. She was one of our several college graduates, and she recognized a phrase of Shakespeare's which Violet used to finish a line: "footsteps in the sands of time." Aida was tough. She was also a leader, but her stridency kept people at bay. In spite of that, or maybe because of it, she could direct the whole group. Sometimes she was the center of a spat that went nowhere and possibly helped to scare some people off. The inspired part was that she got the group to open up by asking soul-searching questions of herself, rather than by telling stories. These questions of hers often sparked a lyric narrative by someone else in the group. Last I heard, Aida was busy performing in a troupe organized by the young man who recited the first poem of *God's Trombones* at our first workshop.

The afternoon sessions were a different story. I'd been warned that seniors didn't care as much for the afternoons, that they tended to be early birds. Indeed, by the third week, the hot afternoons found our little group holding on with only two regulars and one "sometimer," compared with half a dozen regulars in the morning. One time it seemed as if no one at all would come, but just as I was leaving, Josephine Armstrong arrived, so that there was never a time when I found myself completely deserted. The despondency that resulted from being left alone is not to be underestimated; and even a small group, though not as bad, can be demoralizing. When David Watkins or Josephine was the only person with me, I sensed an uneasiness on his or her part, as well as mine—a disappointment that they should have me all to themselves as if something were being wasted. Maybe they sensed some frustration on my part, intensified since these two never wrote until Josephine unleashed a score of poems at the very end of our sessions. I might add that the pressure I put on myself to produce was intensified by the smallness of the group and their lack of writing, and it probably greatly spurred me to transcribe poems from their speech.

The intimacy that developed from such personal encounters was the flip side of the coin and allowed for some real heart-and-soul talks, which in turn made for interesting transcriptions.

Josephine was the only ''junior'' in the classes. She wanted to know if she could come to the workshop even though she wasn't a senior. She was only forty-six. As if to justify her inclusion in the group, she added that she had asthma bad enough to get a disability check because she couldn't work; this was ''sort of being retired.''

Asthma

I'm off the injections.
Now I'm taking Vanceril.
I used to take too much.
They put me on Prednis
& they weaned me off Prednis.
I've taken Isoprel
but it was enlarging my stomach.
Now I'm taking a Terbutaline
tablet every eight hours.
If I discontinue I'd probably
end up in the emergency room.

She's the one I think of most, the one I feel I failed the most, because in some ways she had lived the least and could have gained the most from me. Toward her I was very sympatico in that I saw many foreshadowings of things I had always feared. She'd started off great. Got out of high school with excellent marks and took courses at a college in nearby Montgomery, Alabama. She did well, borrowed a little, and enrolled in a professional women's college in

Florida. Toward the end of the year her father died, and she had to go home and help out. She got a job in the school at Woody, Alabama, and taught all the subjects, all the grades, all ten or twelve kids for several years, and then because of murky dealings that seemed ultimately to swivel on the stool of honor, Josephine spoke her mind and was fired.

In our dialogues I learned much of her story. She wasn't apt to talk about her past unless I asked. She was well informed and often talked about the news, world events, geography. Geography actually led me to a new take on our conversations.

When I realized that Josephine had lived in Montgomery all through the sixties, I surmised that her interest in politics insured a special feeling for the great hero, Martin Luther King. Maybe, I thought, she had even seen the man. When I mentioned his name she began: "I went to his church." She knew I was writing down what she said, and she really played it up for me with great dignity, building momentum, using all the things I'd talked about—contracts, metaphors, even internal rhyme.

"Everybody was surprised that the people would follow him—the old, the young, the maids, and the aids. Because it was rough . . ." As if this conversation had been a catalyst, the next week she brought in several quasi-political poems, and the week after, a bunch more. She also wrote a handful of very personal demi-eulogies to her family. It seemed all very freeing. These writings seemed to justify something in her life to herself, justify in the typesetting sense even, making a clean edge.

It was appropriate that Josephine and David should be the principal members of the afternoons, in light of their longstanding political involvement. To complement Josephine's work with Dr. King, David had stories to tell about Marcus Garvey proudly leading a hundred thousand people up Lenox Avenue. He suggested I read Mencken and Cowley. He told me how hard he had worked to get Blacks jobs on the buses and subways. His involvement had not become restricted with age. He was an active member of a library friends' group doing vital neighborhood work. He shared small newsletters with me. David didn't really write any of his own ideas or stories down, which may have led him to talk more, giving me more chances to write them down, which I did. In fact, his only writing effort in the entire five months was four skillfully playful stanzas arguing how memory is too tricky to be relied on for writing.

When, on some days, both David and Josephine showed up, we had informed geopolitical discussions. We debated the pros and cons of late capitalism, and we speculated on Kremlin dictates. We reviewed the lives of writers too, Baldwin in Paris, Dunbar in Harlem, Malcolm X in Mecca. David, Josephine, and myself shared a great deal.

IV

Having never taught a workshop, much less a cross-cultural one, I petitioned suggestions from Ted Berrigan, a poet who has taught in many different situations. It had been my unarticulated design to evoke the fantastic, the circus aspects, Christmas and other holidays. Ted backed off this approach, unindulgently amused.

"Oh no, no, you want to aim for the familiar, the everyday. Have them write about what was in their house, what was on the radio and on people's lips after dinner had been cleared up, what was the dog's name, who won the pennant. Have them describe their walk to school. It was probably a good distance and that's something they had to do every day in all different seasons."

This, combined with the religious background of all the workshop members, led me to introduce the church in childhood as appropriate subject matter. The writings that ensued, based on early church experiences, were marvelously akin to each other. The particulars of the white dress, the big pink bow in the clean hair, the warnings not to get dirty—all these elements were either present in each member's work or were recognized in the work of others. This similarity of culture provided a strong basis for group cohesion. Having begun to solidify the group, I could then really turn my attention to content, to what we were going to examine in our writings and what models we would use.

A group must be cohesive to endure any strong, spirited debates about, say, literary taste or politics or race. Before introducing controversy, it is good to bind the group by emphasizing cultural and historical similarities which show how its members have all lived through kindred trials and triumphs.

One of my chief problems was to steer between those naturally inclined toward verse and those geared toward prose. At first I switched from week to week, but soon the prospect of five months worth of quasi-random subject selection seemed awesome to me.

My method was generally to introduce writings that seemed pertinent to the previous week. More often than not this presentation was oriented toward subject rather than structure. For example, early on I brought in prose poems by Juan Ramon Jimenez to bridge the prose-poetry chasm. I chose poems about New York City because my stress was on detail and content more than form.

I told Marc Kaminsky about this dilemma concerning prose and poetry and group unity and asked for some advice in regard to content. Sensing the frenzy that might accompany the successive weeks of sequential assignments, Marc gave me an idea for a single, overall plan of attack. In keeping with many of the members who professed interest in autobiography, Marc suggested a plan based on the life history of the individual. Each week we would simply move from one phase to the next of an individual's life. We started with childhood and proceeded to adolescence; then on to marriage, bearing children, finding work, etc. I was grateful to Marc for providing an idea for this overall approach because I felt it freed me of the burden of developing a whole new assignment every week. Now I had something to fall back on. Dividing life like this, roughly into "life stages," allowed me to bring in appropriate literature and helped weld the group together by unifying the focus of their writing.

Another bonus of chronological biography was that, once set in motion and running smoothly, it provided me with a theme I could use to focus the workshop conversation when it diverged too widely from our now apparent goal. After three weeks, when the chronological overview was operating under its own steam and the question of whether to concentrate on prose assignments or poetry was resolved by each member, I turned to another issue relevant to working with the elderly. The fundamental issue we had to answer was: whether to write about the past or about the present. So, as soon as I felt confident, I reintroduced day-to-day writing. I actually gave a double assignment each week. First they were to write of the appropriate stage in their life, and second, I supplied models that would stimulate present-tense creation. To my delight, several members usually would be moved to do both assignments. The autobiography generally was presented in page-long prose blocks, and the current daily pieces were shaped by line breaks and stanzas.

The autobiographical approach worked well for most people. One woman had a poetic sensibility that excelled in brief, emotional lyrics and balked at the seeming infinity of prose. In an effort to bond her lyrical quality with a subject of more duration than a few lines, I suggested she write a eulogy. In a final burst of writing, this woman wrote a piece entitled "Tribute to Pop" in which she evoked a wonderful man who brought his daughters oysters and potatoes at night before he went to work at the Winter Garden.

At a typical meeting each member would read his or her latest "homework" to the class, and the others would respond in turn; or if need be, I would draw out conversation by my own comments or by asking someone in particular how he or she felt about a certain aspect of the work. More often than not, especially as the weeks progressed and a familiarity was established, the comments would come like gasps of recognition:

"Oh—we bleached our clothes on rocks, too!"

"We had a huge red bow above the fireplace at Christmastime, too"

"We got firecrackers in our stockings, too."

"You must have lived in Georgia, too."

From the start, I had been scribbling down these concurrences, the inserted tales and accounts from the past, their reflections and resolves. (This came to be the source of a third or so of the material printed in *Over The Years*.) The speed at which I had to write to keep up with people's speech served two very important functions that effectively changed many of the "sayings" from documentation into real poems. To begin with, writing as fast as I could made the lines on the paper disappear, the letters grew and clustered toward the middle of the page, foreshortening the lines. The velocity of natural talk left no time for me to reflect on the fine points such as where or when to break the line or add periods or commas; but because we do talk very rhythmically and metrically, the breaks sort of "fell out" by themselves. The other vital aspect that attached itself to this fast clip was a slight economy that played in and out, like a fish sometimes tautens the line and sometimes lets it out. It was so important to keep up with the speaker that there wasn't time for some articles or conjunctions to be written down. Somehow, combined with line breaks and the reality of unself-conscious conversation, this process worked thoroughly well.

I got so intrigued I began to introduce topics to see if they would respond, to see if the right topic among these friends could galvanize their language, make it rustproof. And remember, they were not talking for the pen madly transcribing their words, they were talking to each other—listening and being part of a living conversation. One of the tenets I referred to in the workshops was "you write like you talk," but they never actually did this. Their writings were different from their talk. They were really more skilled at talking. I did not fully confront them with the fact that I was making poems out of their talk until nearly the end. This meant their language kept its accuracy and scope.

Yet subliminally I think they knew what I was up to, and perhaps this unfocused knowledge played an important part in the words they chose about the topic, the pride or honesty and care conveyed at the instant of word selection. In this kind of poem, they talked and I wrote, that was all. I offered no resistance or direction. Usually these pieces would spin off from a poem someone read. Someone else would make a comment, maybe another person would comment too or relate an account. These poems are very innocent, although this one, "Sewing," is the least so.

I might add that this method didn't always work so well.

Sewing

That's my line
But you could have 3 times
that much money & not work
half as hard

I enjoy it
I like it
It's not work for me
But I don't like to be pressured
That's why I went into being
a sample hand because you didn't have to rush

Piece work you have to rush
to make a piece
If it's piece work you're working
it's too fine, needle fine—Mamie Walker, Helen Bonaparte,
    & Violet J. Campbell

When, in the final sessions, I showed people what I had written while they spoke, they were astonished.

"Did I say this?"

"Did you write this?"

"This is better than I could ever write, are you kidding?!"

"But they are your words, yours and mine," I said, referring as well to my authorial pride and understanding of their words. For this process was really two-way. It took my ears to "hear" the poem lurking within their spoken speech. I provided the acknowledgment necessary to release it and the recognition to know what they were saying. It was a genuine collaboration between a professional poet and a native/intuitive poet.

After I shared some of these collaborative poems with them, there were only enough sessions left for us to attempt in-class collaborations a couple of times. These collaborations between the workshop members were much less "fused" than pieces by a single author; they could be tampered with and they could stand the impact of wholesale revision. The slight hint of competition, the gamelike give-and-take of throwing lines back and forth really challenged us all. It made us step out a little. David and Josephine became humorous and inventively cynical in their poem, "Politics."

Politics

Politics is like a fish without a bicycle.
Politics is a man with a mask.
Politics is Nero applying for fire insurance.
Politics is a basketball court in Harlem.
I think of politics as a notorious game.
Politics is a yellow lemon
like a yellow brick road.
Politics is promises, promises, promises
kicking donkeys, big elephants.
The problem is if you don't play ball
by the rules. . .
That's when you get in over your head.

The possibility of coaxing or coaching this kind of poem seems more apparent when contrasted with a poem like "Sewing." The following poem, "July," was modeled initially after James Schuyler's "month poems." When Mamie said, "The sun rode the horse," I said "like what," and she created a metaphor, "like a volcano," that extended the original image. Mamie caught on to the idea of extending the image quickly and went on to tell me the rest of the poem. I was very excited by her inventiveness and stature. Again I was powerfully made aware of the honor and importance of leading a workshop.

July

July is a black horse covered in sweat.
Its eyes are ruby shadows.
The sun rides the horse
like a volcano belching its yellow fury.
July the 4th is a bucking bronco—
fireworks, flags, bells tolling
whistles blowing, horns & balloons.
The greatest festival is in July.
She raises high her flags.
People who believe in dreams
believe a black horse is power.
She draws the heavy days
like a curtain
that ends
the romantic play.
July carries all
its belongings.
Even the sun is great.

An incident occurred during the last morning session that I had
anticipated in a way, before the workshops had even begun. I had
met a man, while recruiting members from the churches and centers
in the area, who was curious about autobiography. He paused by a
humming water fountain to lean on his cane, and peering through his
glasses at some obscure vanishing point, he shared a moment of his
life with me. During World War II, Jackie Robinson had been his
friend and his platoon captain. I was excited by his brush with fame
and history and had a premonition that someone in one of my workshops would have a fascinating personal account about a famous
personage.

At that last workshop meeting, we were reading a poem that had
been sent in the mail to the group by a member on vacation. Her
poem about a young man playing basketball at the crossroads of life
was punctuated by the names of black heroes. As one woman read
the poem, Mamie was touched by the mention of the legendary
blues artist, Billie Holliday. As the poem ended, the two women
began to share their memories and impressions of her. My blood felt
prickly and numb at the same time. My ears buzzed like blue neon
as the two women spoke with great affection and sympathy for the
tragic figure. I wrote down their words as they related their en-

counters to each other. The love they showed for this singer, two
decades dead, was expressed in their tones, muted and somber.
Back and forth they went, from one to the other, dipping into the
teeming past.

Billie Holliday

She was a friendly person.
She was a swell person.
She was really loved I think.
She used to live in the 140's.
Then she was downtown—99th,
8 West 99th St.
She was successful but she had
her problems.
She was in so much trouble.
She was arrested & away for a couple of years.
She happened to be making her comeback.
She was on TV & somehow or another
we got tickets.
I was shocked at how she looked
at me.
People said they felt so bad for her.
Some people have a good heart
but they try to do so much for others
they hurt themselves.
Some of the time when she should have been
looking out for herself she would
be thinking of someone else.
I hated to see her go like that.

The people used to come from
downtown with their chauffeurs.
I didn't have the money to buy
a drink in there.
Connie's Inn it was called.
Small's Paradise was a big club.
Connie's was more intimate.
She could sing the blues.
One thing about her career—she kept
climbing as long as she lived.
I don't know if she was living

in a cold water flat then
but I used to go over on some Sunday afternoons.
She told it all on her way out,
"Your life is a gamble—
you might win, you might lose."—Mamie Walker
   & Helen Bonaparte

As the two women took turns, responding almost sentence for
sentence, Mamie's tough regard resounded movingly against Helen's
misty sentiment. It was a very special moment, I think most of all
for me. Later when I read this poem that I wrote from their conversation, I got chills. Mamie told me before we all said good-bye that
when she had lived on West 99th, while she was in her forties during
the early fifties, she had lived just down the hall from the great
singer. I had gotten what I guess I wanted. It was nothing less than
tapping the legacy.

Heal, Body, Heal:
Invocations to Hope and Health

Rochelle Ratner

1. WORKING WITH CONVALESCENTS—BURKE REHABILITATION CENTER

An island is an oasis
An oasis in the desert
Burke is one of the finest places I've heard of
Burke is a temple realizing the original Burke's concept
    toward humanity
A Viennese father figure set somewhere in the woods of
    Salzburg
Burke is like a big plate of chicken soup with matzoh
    balls
We have a patient on our floor who's always dreaming of
    cream cheese and bagels
My children come to see me almost every day
    They find it very calm, a soothing motel after a long
    day of hard driving
A sanctuary that takes people from the outside world and
    prepares them to go back into it
Burke is like my electric wheelchair—it gets me all over.
                                              —Group Poem

We pushed two round tables together in the small secondfloor library. The recreation therapists went off to help bring in the participants, most of whom were in wheelchairs and needed assistance. I sat at the table and felt sort of helpless. I was used to working with people of this age in senior centers, but I sensed that these people

85

were different. In a senior center I've heard women complain that they find it difficult to walk far; the woman I now saw pulling up close to the table did not have to complain, it was obvious that she needed help getting out of her wheelchair. I understood that we were going to be dealing here with feelings that were still raw. Most of the participants had never written before and were not accustomed to using literary form as a mask for what they found difficult to say directly. I recognized that these workshops would play a crucial part in the lives that some of the participants would lead from here on.

At this first session there was one participant, Jeff, who seemed barely able to move, let alone write. When we passed out paper, I simply worked around him. Then one of the recreation therapists saw him scribbling at a piece of tape on the arm of his chair and shoved paper in front of him. He wrote something like "I am Jeff," and even this was received with encouragement. The patients and staff were teaching me the way things were done at Burke.

I tried several different writing ideas and over the various work-shops developed four lessons which seemed to follow a definite progression yet were basic enough for new participants at any session to follow. During the first series of workshops, I spent the fourth session focusing on "prayers." We spoke of prayer as a form of direct address, an asking, which could be directed at anyone. We discussed the difference between "prayer" and "blessing." Yet most of the poems dealt with sickness, the need to be healed. They asked for healing.

I should have known. In the month since I had begun teaching there, I had found my own poems moving toward a definition of sickness and health. These workshops would be of value only if they could help the participants come to terms with their illness and the health that still remained.

I began to see growth in people from week to week. At the third session we had confronted illness directly in "talking to a part of the body"; at the fourth and final session, one of the women picked up on that theme and described what the experience of attending these workshops had meant for all of us:

Heal, Body, Heal

What have I done to you to justify what you
have done to me, all unknowingly?
Tell me, can you heal as well as destroy?

If so, how?
If so, tell me—I shall do
as you say.—Florence O'Brien

2. THE WORKSHOPS

The workshops would begin around 7:30 in the evening, but we seldom started writing before 8:00. I made sure that paper and pencils were available, but they were not passed out until it came time to write. I stressed that no one had to write if he or she did not want to; they were welcome to join in anyway and listen or participate in the conversation. And many participants did just that. Others, who insisted they couldn't write, would begin to scribble once they saw other people working. Some patients would get visitors and leave in the middle of the session; other times the visitors joined in; other patients got tired and decided to leave. We tried to keep things as loose and relaxed as possible. In general, the workshops were over by 9:00, though sometimes conversations continued.

At the first workshop we went around the table and introduced ourselves. Going around again, I asked each person to "tap out the rhythm of your first name on the table, emphasizing the number of syllables, which syllable is accented, whether the rhythm is slow or fast." If there was a patient who did not seem able to move his or her arms, I adapted the exercise by asking everyone either to tap out the rhythm or hum it. Someone challenged me: "What does all this have to do with writing?" The answer came before I could fully think it out: "Poetry is rhythm, and concentrating on our names, the most personal part of ourselves, is directly related to what the poem should do." I read some poems in which poets had dealt with the meaning and sound of their names.

Rachel

(Rachel—ra'chel—an ewe)
We named you
for the sake
of the syllables
and for the small boat
that followed the *Pequod*,
gathering lost children

of the sea.
We named you
for the dark-eyed girl
who waited at the well
while her lover
worked seven years
and again
seven.
We named you
for the small daughters
of the Holocaust
who followed their six-pointed stars
to death
and were all of them
known as
Rachel.—Linda Pastan

Rosemary

Rosemary.
    Rosemary Hughes.
        Rosemary Hughes Ramos
      Rosemary Hughes Ramos Daniell
Rosemary Hughes Ramos Daniell Coppelman.
    Rosemary Hughes Ramos Daniell
      Rosemary Hughes Ramos
    Rosemary Hughes
Rosemary who's?
    Rosemary's.—Rosemary Daniell

We talked about the importance of names in the Old Testament. In Genesis 17, for example, God says: "No longer shall your name be Abram [that is, *exalted father*], but your name shall henceforth be Abraham [*father of a multitude*], for I have made you father of a multitude of nations." Or, in Genesis 25, Rebekah is described giving birth to twins: "Afterward his brother came forth, and his hand had taken hold of Esau's heel; so his name was called Jacob [that is, *He takes by the heel* or *He supplants*]."

We discussed superstitions and religious traditions regarding naming, such as the Jewish belief that the soul of a dead person does not come to rest until its name has been given to an infant, or the custom of changing the name of a sick child: thus was the Angel of

Death confused when he came for Jacob and found Seth. I brought
in a dictionary of names and read the meaning of each person's
name. This, in itself, was instrumental in sparking off images for
some participants:

Matthew

What God gave him.
God gave me a good life. In all my
troubles he was there to help me. Even
in my trouble now: I am an old man
and he helped me to recuperate fast from
my heart operation—Matthew Kaftan

Barbara—the stranger
Strange to me or strange to others?
Am I strange to myself?
Do I know me?
What is my rhythm
Or do I mean my bio-rhythm?

Does he know me—the stranger?
Does he understand the stranger in me?
I have often wondered to myself
Do I know me—do you know me?

Are we strangers to each other?
Are we now less strange as the years flow by?
Has life brought us closer?
I wonder—more and more as I think of us—
of you, of me.—Barbara Willig

For other participants, thinking of their names sparked off childhood memories. Billie, who wrote the following poem, mentioned
that she had not thought about her lost name since she was a young
child.

Libby, they say she called me,
Libelleh, my Mom.
I don't remember ever being
called Libelleh, you see I was only two
and she had already left us.
She was thirty four and her name was Sara.

No one ever called me Libelleh after
she was gone.
Now I am "Billie"—I sure
would like to hear the name Libelleh.
Now I am Billie, full grown, and
never to hear the name Libelleh again.

I came away from that first workshop with a feeling that I had suc-
ceeded in giving each person his or her own name back. And along
with that went the strong affirmation of individuality: many people
were looking at themselves as if for the first time.

Barbara Willig, who'd written the "stranger" poem earlier that
evening, was able to take the theme of "name as identity" one step
further. This time she was able to make the name into an image:

Super giant—I was always big.
At least I always felt so big:
Big hands, big feet,
I always envied my little friends.

It was not until I grew up a bit
I could stand tall and not feel so big.
I learned words like regal and Junoesque.

They made me feel more desirable.
They gave me a new self image.
I was no longer a super-giant,
Perhaps only a giant—but a nice one.

"Super Giant" was actually the name of a flower. Over the summer, I'd been glancing at a Burpee Seed Catalogue and was fascinated by some of the names for different flowers. Without telling
people what the flower was, I read some of the names: Summer
Sun, Plum Pudding, Majorette, Christmas Pepper, Blue Fairy Tale,
Organ Pipe, Native's Comb. I asked them to write about the flower,
what it looked like, how it got its name, or whatever else one of the
names called to mind. We talked about how people in a hospital are
always receiving gifts of flowers and discussed ways they could
relate the names to themselves.

Barbara's two poems had revealed an openness about herself
which interested me. I was anxious to find out more about her and
wheeled her back to her room that night so we would have a chance

to talk. She told me she had always promised herself that she would someday find the time to write, but had continually put it off. I pointed out that she had the time now. During the next three sessions I was continually encouraging her to try some writing on her own during the day, but she kept insisting she didn't feel well enough, she wanted to be at home before she really started writing on her own. After leaving Burke, Barbara joined a writing workshop at a senior center near her home.

At the second session, I wanted to give participants a form that would allow them to write about their concerns without being "personal." The key seemed to be in the use of images. I asked each of them to "write about yourself as if you were an animal or an object." I took care to make sure that the examples I read had a happy, playful feeling, such as David Ignatow's "The Bagel":

> I stopped to pick up the bagel
> rolling away in the wind
> annoyed with myself
> for having dropped it
> as if it were a portent.
> Faster and faster it rolled,
> with me running after it
> bent low, gritting my teeth,
> and I found myself doubled over
> and rolling down the street
> head over heels, one complete somersault
> after another like a bagel
> and strangely happy with myself.

Whatever animal or object they chose to be, I wanted them actually to *become* it. "If you're a floor, is it because people walk all over you? What does it feel like? Are you wood, linoleum, or is there a carpet over you? Do children run barefoot across you? This poem by John Haines does an excellent job of imagining precisely what it feels like to be a cauliflower":

The Cauliflower

> I want to be a cauliflower,
> all brain and ears,
> meditating on the origin of gardens
> and the divinity of Him

who carefully binds my leaves.

With my blind roots touched
by the songs of the worms
and my rough throat throbbing
with strange vegetable sounds,
perhaps I'd feel the parting stroke
of a butterfly's wing. . .

Not like those cousins the cabbages,
whose heads, tightly folded,
see and hear nothing of this world,
dreaming only of the yellow
and green magnificence
that is hardening within them.

We spoke of how poetry permits you to become any animal or object you want to be, simply by imagining yourself as that. No one could criticize your fantasies. And yet my reaction to Max Kornweitz's poem was to want to cry out, "You've got more than this!" He had seemed calm and quiet. The poem shows his acceptance of illness as just one more thing he was fated to endure:

I think of myself as a small horse,
Hard-working, always sleepy,
Who looks like he's carrying all the hardship
     of life on his back
And never gets a break to enjoy a better life,
Who is always tired, and looks for a place to relax.

I sensed that Charlotte Stern had begun writing her poem from much the same point of view that we saw in Max's poem. The first two lines lead us to believe she will go on to talk about things that happened to her which she would have liked to forget. But perhaps writing those lines acted as a catharsis for her—she saw them written there and realized that no, she didn't want to forget, she just wanted to remember the happier times:

I am an elephant.
I wish I could not have a memory, and forget.
However it has sometimes been a good point
Because I don't forget nice things I experienced.

So I try to concentrate on positive things
To make life easier for me and those around me.

Charlotte understood that during this period of illness she would
need people around to help her and care for her; Doris Silverstein
took that one step further. Her poem is ambivalent: she sees friends
and the care they offer as a threat as well as a comfort. Like Max
Kornweitz, she was coming to an acceptance of her life. Illness was
forcing her to look at everything around her in much more personal
terms; she watched the flowers wilt in her room and realized it
would be possible for her to wilt as well. As she watched the flowers
struggling to survive, the struggle her own body was going through
became that much clearer to her.

I feel like a bunch of flowers.
I like being flowers and yet I am afraid
Of all the people who will come and pick me—
Petal by petal.
I want to stay whole and yet I know that someone,
Many people, will want to take part of me with them.
My petals are getting less and less.
The water that is nurturing me is evaporating
I would like at this moment to be in a florist's case—
Cool, well cared for—
And to stay fresh and lovely and alive for longer
Than is possible for a flower's lifetime.

There were other people who already had a strong sense of who
they were, and for them the use of images seemed too much of a
bother. Anna Weintraub wanted to be precisely what she was, and
her poem is a beautiful affirmation of that. It becomes almost an ode
to the recuperative powers of the body:

I am 82
     Still going strong
Broke my hip
     Still going strong
Had it mended
     And still going strong
     You can't keep a woman like me down.

Anna's poem led us directly into the third session: an affirmation

that the body *can* recuperate. I had found that people seemed to ig-
nore the injured parts of their bodies, rather than really work on
them. I told them that "the body can recuperate, but you have to *tell
it what you want.* People talk to plants, and we're told they grow
better. Why shouldn't the body, or one part of the body, react the
same way?"

The workshop happened to coincide with Valentine's Day, so naturally discussion centered on the heart. Some pointed out that the
physical therapist was constantly reminding her that "the heart is a
muscle" and must be used to produce movement. We wrote the following group poem, passing around a sheet of paper with each person writing, then folding it over so the next person couldn't see what
had already been written:

The Heart

The heart is a muscle
The heart has become a geographical designation:
Heart of the nation, tobacco country, etc.
The heart beats and is measured by machines
But not when we use the word to mean "feelings"
The heart is a pump sending blood through our veins
The heart reflects the glory of the sun
Hearts made of chocolate and other goodies
Hearts made of muscle and blood
Chocolate hearts are good to eat
Muscle and blood hearts are hard to treat
The heart is the symbol of love and
The maintainer of life
The heart beats the rhythm of living and loving
The heart is a very delicate organ, so please do not
        break mine.

This poem has a marked tendency toward cliché and abstraction. I
saw that writing *about* a part of the body could easily lead to senti-
mentality, which was one of the reasons I wanted people to *address*
the body. I told them to "be as specific as possible. Don't try to talk
to your entire body, but choose one part, and tell it precisely what
you want from it. If you can give the reader a clear picture of that
one part, he will have no trouble imagining the rest of your body.
It's like a moment caught in a snapshot." We made a few small mir-
rors available, in case they wanted to write about a part of the body

they couldn't see otherwise, but no one bothered to use them. Perhaps they were all too aware of their physical conditions; they wanted to use the poem to lift them above everyday reality:

> My forehead is wrinkled.
> I would like it to be smooth.
> Someday I will plant
> something there. . . (anonymous)

It took me a long time to find a poem I could use as an example which would force participants into a direct encounter with their bodies and handicaps, yet at the same time would not present a completely negative focus. The poem I finally selected is by Robert Winner, himself a paraplegic:

> To My Face, after Illness
>
> From your bones on out
> you give the lie to suffering.
> You ought to be more lined with pain.
> You should give a stronger impression
> in photographs
> of the heartbreak caged in your fat.
>
> Mess of tissues!
> Maybe I should be grateful to you
> for remembering,
> for leaving printed on this flesh—
> its sun-tanned jowls—
> these inescapable paragraphs
> which tell the original story.

After hearing this, David Gordon dictated to me the following poem:

> My left hand and arm,
> like a lover,
> always beside me,
> always to help me—
> you burn me up
> because my right
> is not as strong as my left.

But then the one time you disappoint me
and become numb to my flesh,
I don't even know you're there.
Then I look down
and I expect to see
a bare stomach
but instead I see you.
It comes to mind
how I have no fury
like a woman scorned.
The swan has turned into an ugly duckling
for what once was really beautiful
to me
has become an appendage,
like a lobster claw:
red, raw, and mean-looking,
with no help
but just ugliness.
To see and to feel
and not to see and not to feel. . .
a paradox.
To think I always took care of you,
but when I really needed you
you were never there,
and you never took care of me.

David insisted he'd never written before, yet everything he dictated, and the speed at which he was able to progress from image to image, belied that assertion. While writing this, he had trouble remembering the word "paradox," and made me look in two dictionaries and a thesaurus in order to find it.

David himself was a paradox; nothing else he said gave any hint of the anger he expressed in this poem. He contributed a lot to every conversation and showed an interest in everyone who spoke. I remember one night the recreation therapists were discussing a trip with patients to a local movie theater, and he mentioned that he would not want to go with them: "People around here know me, and I'd rather they didn't see me yet."

Kathleen Cudney, like David, was angry at her body. She had every right to be. She was in her early twenties; arthritis was slowly crippling her completely. (The younger patients were in a different unit of the hospital, and many of their activities were separated from those of the older patients, but I wanted the workshops open to everyone and found it easier to relate at first to the two patients closer to my own age.) At the first session, Kathi seemed to be sullen, but as the sessions progressed she gradually opened up. The first poem she wrote she refused to share with the group. I read it and immediately perceived that she had written before. The hospital staff told me there were anxious to find activities that could interest her now that her physical capacity was more limited, and writing seemed an important step in developing other interests.

At the third session she brought in some of her old poems, many of which she was now revising. During this workshop she wrote an angry poem to her body, and she read it. David's poem had already been read, and perhaps that influenced her. But she heard other participants read more encouraging poems, thanking injured parts of their bodies for the good times they had shared and promising that those times would come again. While we were sitting around talking, after reading the poems, she began to write again, rewriting the same poem with an entirely different emphasis.

1.

My right hand
serves me no more—
now to write
I must use both.
Time consuming.
My legs serve me poorly
or not at all;
muscle strength
is gone.
My head
serves me no more—
Jumbled thoughts,
mixed-up feelings,
confusion.

2.

Right hand
why do you fail me?
I always took good care

of you,
kept you as warm
as I could in winter,
even if
I had to sit on you.
Sorry if it hurt,
but it hurt more
when you were cold.
At least I tried.
Why don't you
try harder?
You can do it,
I know you can,
so let's keep going, trying,
together.

In the first poem, Kathi dealt with three separate parts of her body: her right hand, her legs, and her head. The second poem proved that, with a little effort, she *did* have the ability to concentrate and focus on only one part, as if at the same time she was healing the "jumbled thoughts" of the first poem.

Kristin Maher was a lot like Kathi. She was also an arthritic patient, and she was younger than most of the others—I'd say probably in her mid- to late thirties. She was able to begin writing at each session without any prompting; aside from reading her work she was fairly quiet. But here the resemblances stopped. Everything she wrote was from a very positive point of view, and her poems usually focused more on other people than herself. In speaking to her body, she dealt with the part that she felt put her in the closest touch with others.

Ears,
Thank you for bringing me music
Which, depending on which type,
Brings peace or a livelier gaiety.
And ears, through you come
Voices of friends or birds,
My cats,
Kind people, brusque voices
And then music
Which closes the circle of love.

Kristin's poem started me thinking. It now struck me that when you talk to someone this directly, you expect an answer. What would happen if we took the theme of sickness and health and started to look at it as a dialogue between the body and the mind? "If we can talk this directly to a part of the body, it's only right for *it* to be able to give its version." When I first suggested that people now write an answer to their first poem, I was expecting something more or less humorous. Yet the only people who wrote humorous answers were the two recreation therapists and myself. Kristin's second poem is remarkable in its ability to endow her ears with as much kindness for "her" as she originally felt for "them":

> Yes, we heard you.
> What we have given
> Is safely in storage,
> So that even if we stopped hearing
> You wouldn't.
> The music will still be there
> Even when we and the rest of you
> Aren't.

Later, when I typed Kristin's poem, I realized that she used these words to assuage her fear of death. And certainly death was an imminent presence for all the people in these workshops. Yet I kept pushing it from my mind. The prospect of my own death was something I did not want to face, and I felt it was necessary to continue the workshops as if others had not faced it either. There seemed to be an unspoken agreement that no one would destroy my illusions. Everyone listened politely to my suggestions for assignments, then they went ahead and wrote the poems they felt they had to write. In having a part of the body "answer" the poem addressed to it, they had turned an exercise I had seen as playful into a profoundly significant dialogue. Not one poem consciously fought the assignment I had given; the participants simply added their own content to the form I provided.

There were similar results with an exercise triggered by Denise Levertov's marvelous poem, "The Wings":

> Something hangs in back of me,
> I can't see it, can't move it.

I know it's black,
a hump on my back.

It's heavy. You
can't see it.

What's in it? Don't tell me
you don't know. It's

what you told me about—
black

inimical power, cold
whirling out of it and

around me and
sweeping you flat.

But what if,
like a camel, it's

pure energy I store,
and carry humped and heavy?

Not black, not
that terror, stupidity

of cold rage; or black
only for being pent there?

What if released in air
it became a white

source of light, a fountain
of light? Could all that weight

be the power of flight?
Look inward: see me

with embryo wings, one
feathered in soot, the other

blazing ciliations of ember, pale
flare-pinions. Well—

could I go
on one wing,

the white one?

I thought it would be interesting if people could "invent a new part of their bodies." We talked about science fiction and the way it makes use of this device. If we were to invent a new part, then it would most likely be a natural extension of the parts we already have. And certainly we had a lot of fun talking about the possibilities. But the poems were once again down to earth and practical. Several people, many of whom were stroke patients, wrote about inventing new brains.

> I would like to invent a brain
> That healthily lasts 80 years
>   and then immediately stops with no pain.
> This would alleviate much
>   unnecessary suffering and heartbreak.
> White as an angel
> And just as trusting—Mr. S.

When he wrote this poem, Mr. S. was an active participant in all the workshops. He was able to get around without much trouble, but was constantly complaining that his mind would not let him pronounce the word he wanted. He seemed to be continually reaching for something and then giving up. When my eyes caught his for a moment, I had the feeling that he knew something I didn't know. It didn't matter that outwardly he seemed to be getting better, inwardly he was dying, and he knew it. When I came back to Burke for another series of workshops, two or three months later, he had returned as a patient. He did not come to the workshops this time. The recreation therapists told me they were no longer able to get him to participate in anything, and after a few weeks he was transferred to a nursing home.

It was out in the open now; we talked about the fact that he was dying. Once I accepted that, the poem he had written about "inventing a new part of the body" took on deeper meaning. And looking again over the poems he wrote, I found another one—written earlier that same evening—which captures that same sense of finality. He was not able to focus on any one part of his body, and he was not able to talk to it either. He stated simply what he felt; actuality became a dream of the future without his being aware of it:

> What have I done to my body?
> Abused it,

Amused it,
Busted it many times.
This is a never-ending game.
And then the ball game is over
It stops abruptly,
And peace will be eternal.

In the first three sessions, I had guided the participants through an assertion of individuality, the transferring of their feelings onto an object, and a direct encounter with their illness. Now I wanted them to write a *healing poem*, and I read some primitive healing poems as examples:

Prayer to Heal a Sick Child

O white chicken, good chicken,
chicken that is just a chick, crying peep-peep,
Throw off, shed away Bale Oke, spirit of sores,
Bale Pali, spirit of sudden bad changes.
Release sickness from the body, from inside the body
where it has gone deep, deaf to our call—
O white chicken, good chicken,
chicken that is just a chick, crying peep-peep.
Sickness, follow the pig, the male pig
to the end of the mountain,
to the end of the valley, to the end of the mountainslope,
to the end of the steep slope on the mountain.
Beat the air from out of, get rid of, release—
your rhinoceros hornbill—
beat the air from out of, get rid of
the sickness from the body;
break its hold on this life. (from the Sarawak Museum Journal,
    translation by Carol Rubenstein)

People seemed confused by the poem. I stopped and just asked them directly: "If I told you to write a *healing poem*, what would you think of?" Talk led to prayer, to doctors, operations, and the simple kindness of nurses. We even somehow got talking about levitation. We spoke of the psychological elements involved in the healing process, how the "laying-on of hands" could be related to the touch of any doctor. We talked about exorcism, where the sickness is ordered out of the body and into some object or animal. I related this to the Old Testament understanding of the scapegoat. I said that people unable to understand what an illness actually is frequently personified it and prayed to it, such as prayers to "Verminus" for the relief from worms. One poem by a contemporary American poet, Rose Drachler, seemed to illustrate my point perfectly—and it was a poem they had no trouble understanding.

Amulet Against Cancer

Big Black dog
who lives away from masters

I growl back at you
Wild dog with no master

I advance slowly
One step at a time

I hit you between the ears
On top of the head

With a wooden spoon
I spit in your face

Then feed you
You must learn to live in my house

In a corner. You must learn
How to live in my house
With me

Florence O'Brien's poem, "Heal, Body, Heal" was written at this session.

Not every participant was able to write, or even talk, directly from their feelings. Sometimes, an exalted sense of poetic language got in the way, as in this poem:

Heal, heal, oh heal
You vast and shapeless depths
Of universal night—
You starry nebulae—
And O, you infinitely small,
You corpuscles of nerve and blood,

You atoms of uranium,
Mercury and sulphur,
And O, you in-between,
You powers of man
By this incantation
Heal, heal, Oh heal!—Mr. D.

Mr. D. was a stroke patient, and at the previous sessions was wheeled in on a stretcher. It was hard for him to see other people and thus get the general mood of the group, so he would talk on endlessly and expect others to listen. At the second session, when we wrote about being an object or an animal, he began with: "It would be nice to be God." This healing poem, for all its faults, was the first poem he had written rather than dictated. He was sitting at the table; for the first time he was joining the group.

When I look back on these workshops, Socrates Vavoudis is one of the people I think about with affection. His father was a Greek poet. In his late fifties, Socrates was still working as a computer engineer, but he had taken writing courses in college and had grown up with literature, I met him standing outside the library door before the second session, and we started talking. There was a calmness and certainty in his presence that made me think he was one of the staff. No, he had had heart surgery.

At the workshop sessions he began writing immediately, but at the final session he was having trouble. At one point I whispered: "If you're stuck, try starting with nonsense syllables and see where that leads you." Though he didn't take my advice, he began writing just after that. He was the last person in the room to begin, but he finished ahead of most of the others.

As soon as he finished writing, he got up and walked around the room for a few minutes. He stepped out into the hall, came back to the table. We were going around the table and reading our poems and came to where he was sitting. He asked us to continue reading and come back to his poem later. He said he was feeling pain. He tols us the assignment had upset him by forcing him to focus on his sickness. When he first came back into the room his hand had been lightly resting on his chest, a gesture common to those with a heart condition. The next poem we heard had an incantational quality to it, and Socrates commented on how soothing our voices were. He sat down, relaxed now. Though I had used this "healing poem" assignment with other groups, this was the first time that everyone

explains: the traditionalists alienate the oppressed
by showing them the world as their enemy; the moderni-
zers alienate them by means of supporting mere reformism
and preserving the status quo.[13]

A (pseudo) "liberating education" in this context
is conceived of in individualistic terms, as something
which belongs to the conscience of the person to be
transformed or converted. The socio-historical praxis
is not duly considered. Freire insists that Christians
ought to get rid of any illusory dream of trying to
change individuals without touching the world they live
in and that the programs for action based on that illusory dream will necessarily be paternalistic and--
quoting Niebuhr--"falsely generous."[14]

Freire believes and warns that religion in Latin
America is moving in this modernizing direction. There
is apparent change in the area of religious practices,
restating of some doctirnal positions and even more
involvement in regard to social, economic and political
problems. However, the measures taken are mere reforms
that fail to produce the radical transformation needed.

c. Social Structures, Consciousness and the
Church. According to Freire's analyses, it is possible
to find interesting correlations between socio-cultural
structures and levels of consciousness which--as stated
in the first chapter--are to be seen in light of historical conditioning. And all this can be related in turn
with the typology of church-religion. This underscores
again the Marxist character of Freire's approach in
which historical-cultural reality is interpreted as a
superstructure in relationship to an infrastructure,
the church. Those levels of consciousness and the
parallel types of religiosity and institutional churches
correspond to the false consciousness concept in the
Marxian analysis. It involves "reification" and alien-
ation because, basically, human experiences and productions are considered as if they were fruits of divine
will written into the nature of cosmic laws. In the
Marxian corrective, human beings are perceived as the
product of a reality which, in fact, was made by actual
human beings, i.e., their historical cultural reality.

In the same connection, the complementarity of
epistemological and theological foundations in Freire's
thought can also be illustrated. We discussed before
the hypothesis that the conscientization process and
method involve the various levels of consciousness and

In his paper "Education, Liberation and the Church," Freire presents a brief characterization of his view of the church, firstly in terms of what he defines as two unfaithful models, as follows.

a. The Traditionalist or Missionary Church. It includes many intensely colonial marks and insists on the "conquering of souls," flight from the "world" and other "necrophilic" attitudes such as the emphasis on sin and hell, the world-heaven dichotomy, the purifying value of suffering in the midst of injustice, debasement of human nature. By the rejection of the world with its "evils" and "vices," a compensation takes place since the "bad world" is in the oppressors' hands: it is a kind of vindication against the owners or rulers of this world.[11]

By having this orientation, the church becomes a refuge for the masses: it is the context and occasion for a "catharsis" which really contributes to further alienate the oppressed because they are separated from the world instead of being helped to confront the social system that destroys the world.[12] Therefore, this church is basically an ally of the ruling classes.

In this religious framework, education is bound to be conditioned by that peculiar vision of the world, faith, human nature and its predicament. The "traditionalist" or "missionary" church can generate only a quietist, alienated and alienating conception of education.

This type of religion that stresses life in the world to come, actually fosters and sanctions closed societies and is instrumental in maintaining the status quo even if it is a state of manifest privation and oppression. For Freire, however, in order to understand and denounce those dynamics, the point of departure for a thorough sociological analysis should be not the religious phenomenon as such, but the structure of the social classes and the class struggle.

b. The "Modern" and "Modernizing" Church. This is the second type of church and religion of which Freire is critical due to their seemingly alienating orientation.

This perspective is really a new version of the traditional church, mainly concerned with the improvement of its instruments of work, and therefore, commited also to the support of the ruling elites. Freire his theological foundations, rather than a precisely formualted conceptual framework.

At this point, our Anabaptist theological perspective must be made explicit.6 It is our thesis that, (1) in spite of the gap existing between Freire's liberation theology and our Anabaptist approach, mutual enrichment can and should take place; (2) emerging from this theological process of critical analysis and constructive reformulation will be an enhanced understanding of creativity itself.

1. Impossible Neutrality

In his interpretation of the church, Freire begins as an educator. That is, he applies to the Christian church and its members the kind of sociological analysis that has illuminated for him the political power and potential of the educational process and institutions. He concludes that if education cannot be neutral, the political non-neutrality of the Christian and the church should, by the same token, never by underestimated.

For Freire, those who proclaim neutrality for the church are either naive in their perception of the church and history, or--intelligently enough--they know how to conceal their real option in favor of the status quo. If they are "naive," they can eventually accept the ideology of domination thereby transforming their "innocence" into "shrewdness." Or else they can renounce to their idealistic illusion of neutrality in a process which implies a kind of Easter (death and resurrection). Renunciation involves the annihilation of several myths cherished by religious people: their "superiority," "purity of heart" and their higher knowledge, their higher position implied in their mission to "save" the poor, the church's presumption of impartiality in its testimony, its theology or its education,7 and so on.

The logic of Freire's critique of pseudoneutrality reads as follows. The defense of "Christianity"--but, actually, the religiously sanctioned ideology that supports the establishment--amounts to the defense of class interests. In the impossible mission of neutrality with regard to the economic-political structures, the church undertakes the task of reconciling the irreconciliable for the sake of "order" and stability. For Freire, a revolutionary person, Christian or not, cannot accept a church which identifies itself with the

oppressive classes, either "naively" or "shrewdly."[8]
In that case, the prophetic function of the church is
suppressed and its testimony, then, means fear of
change and of radical transformation within an unjust
world: the fear of getting lost in the uncertain future.
The Christian church thus becomes "religious," in the
sense of reactionary, attached to tradition as an end
in itself.[9]

In contrast to that picture, Freire refers to the
fate of those faithful Christians who are persecuted
for allegedly contributing to undermine the "Western
and Christian character of our civilization and life-
style." This is particularly the case when the destructive influence of imperialism and neocolonialism is
denounced. For Freire, this is a crude example of the
fact that--in his terms--the "necrophilic" never endure
the presence of the "biophilic." A major task for the
church is, therefore, the denunciation of all injustice
and the announcement of a world less unjust to be built
up by the historico-social praxis on the part of the
oppressed and their strategic allies.

2. Two Types of Unfaithful Church

In his early writings, Freire did not consider the
role of the church in relation to the existing level of
social and political awareness on the part of the
people. He speaks in general terms about "rightist
forces" which oppose social transformation, while count-
ing on the progressive Christian elements--including
priests and bishops--struggling in the direction of a
democratic society and the democratization of culture.
As an educational consultant with the World Council of
Churches, and in the light of further developments in
his thought as already indicated, Freire's criticism
of institutional religion becomes more pointed and
sharper. It appears that his concerns and interests
are then expressed in more explicitly theological terms.
That is to say, his Marxist orientation has become more
apparent and--in parallel fashion--the same has happened
with the religiious inspiration of his social philosophy. This combination is not very surprising given two
interelated phenomena: the relgious-like character of
Marxist ideology and its "theological structure"[10] and
the very nature of Latin American liberation theology
with its heavy reliance on Marxism.

seemed to take the word "healing" as synonymous with "comfort." Socrates' poem expresses that most directly, and he was feeling well enough to read it now:

Healing Senses

Take me oh mother of my senses
and warm me and soothe me.
Absorb all the pain bolts
which must run their course.
Leave me limp with comfort and sleep
to rest in a void of blank security
and warmth.
Let me stay in this posture
at least till I've healed
without new wounds and lightning
bolts of shrieking pain,
and warm me and soothe me.

About Ending

Roland Legiardi-Laura

As usual, the IRT Lex. is running late. The Astor Place station is large and feels larger because there are only a few of us hoping to get somewhere during the mid-afternoon lull. I've read all the posters selling whiskey and the sound of WPLJ. I've studied the graffiti filling the cracks between Linda Ronstadt's teeth. My eyes now linger momentarily on the bas-relief tile beavers adorning the entrance to the platform. For the first time, I note the craft and care taken to make these little fellas. They seem endowed with pride and a fierce devotion to industry, making them fitting symbols for the heart of old Lord Astor's empire, founded, so to speak, on the backs of those creatures. It's a bit ironic that St. Mark's Place, the main artery carrying foot traffic to the Astor Place station, today can boast as its major business secondhand fur stores and punk boutiques selling leather pants.

My pelt fantasy ceases. My stomach is tight. I'm nervous. In one hand I have my tape recorder and notebook, in the other I clutch a small box of Ratner's *hamantashn.* I've never been nervous going to a workshop meeting before, but today's meeting will be our last, and I'm not trekking up to the Bronx as "workshop leader" but rather as a little boy bringing cake to grandma. In this case, when I arrive, there will be four grandmas waiting for me.

The train finally arrives. I lurch into a seat as I and my fellow travelers creak slowly away from the East Village, toward Yankee Stadium. Once the Lex. slides past the fashionable Upper East Side, the ride becomes a rather somber affair, peopled by young mothers and their screaming brood, nodding junkies, street toughs, the elderly, and an assortment of mendicants. The poor begging from the poor.

My trip ends at the Kingsbridge station. The stop is flanked on one side by a row of one-story shops and restaurants and on the other by an immense, still active armory. In the four months that I have been passing this edifice on my way to the Jewish Home and

Hospital, I have not once seen a door or window open, nor have I seen anyone who looks even remotely connected with the military-industrial complex. But the structure itself—a vast tar-capped prone cylinder with an immense brick facade of ramparts, gun turrets and battlements—is very reassuring indeed. No doubt when the Huns come thundering across the rolling plains of Van Cortlandt park, the "Castle" at Kingsbridge will present a formidable obstacle. Perhaps that was the fantasy of those who designed the building for its more insidious purpose of riot control and crowd pacification.

Further up this hill is the home. I am told it is perhaps the best facility of its kind, a large complex of buildings with gardens and a well-manicured front lawn. One enters by way of an automatic sliding door into a large, clean, carpeted lobby. There is always staff and security at the front desk, and everyone is treated politely. I sign in and get a little stick-on visitors' pass. Inwardly I protest but am told that the "residents" feel much safer if everyone is properly identified. Past the desk and around the corner from the main elevator bank is a cluster of offices. It is from one of these offices, small and unmarked, that the social workers and their trainees daily cope with the problems of institutional care of the elderly. It's here that each week I check in with Susan Tye, a social worker and the coleader of the workshop. Today Susan tells me that everyone is upstairs in the lounge waiting, that I should go on ahead and she'll follow in a few minutes. Again more halls. As I pass by the medical offices and dispensary, I am greeted by a long row of faces. I'm special, a visitor. "Someone has a visitor." Their eyes search my features for some clue. To have a visitor is a sign of status at the home. The times I walked this hall with Susan, she was set upon with questions, demands, complaints, entreaties for assistance. It is hard for her, and she has learned to walk fast, to focus her energy rather than dissipate it.

I am struck by the helplessness of the people here. They are mostly in their eighties and nearly all of them have severe health problems. They walk slowly, with pain, have short tempers and have lost the essential dignity that comes with taking care of oneself. Friendships, I imagine, take a long time to develop in such a situation and are often soon betrayed by death. And so it is the social worker who is left the task of dealing with the vast undercurrents of loneliness, abandonment, and rage—undercurrents, because they are almost never directly expressed, but rather appear half-hidden in arguments over petty issues; in squabbles about privacy in the shared living quarters; misunderstandings in the dining hall; cliquish enmities between German and Russian Jews. It becomes difficult, for many impossible, to struggle toward real change at a home. This is it, the last stop. There are no more plans to be made, no new goals to be reached; most of one's friends have died. Perhaps the children and grandchildren will come and visit. . .

A sharp distinction is drawn between the outside world and the "home." Not officially, of course. Passes and leaves are granted without too great restriction, but the urge to go out seems to wane.

What is the point then? To have the old carcass maintained on a per diem basis—for what? So that the progeny may feel a little less guilty or so that society may self-righteously proclaim a creditable exercise of its just will? No matter how fine the facility, no matter how dedicated the staff, there remains this basic flaw: the homes are not real homes. The idea of grouping people together in order to care for them more efficiently has not yet been reconciled with individual dignity and freedom.

I enter the room and am warmly greeted. It seems as if I'm fully prepared for this phase of the workshop, its "ending." Susan and I have been readying everyone for weeks now. We carefully mentioned at the beginning and end of each session how many more meetings were left. We talked about my reasons for ending "this phase" of my work. Even a fortuitous job crisis, when for a time I thought I would be laid-off prematurely, thus ending the class sooner than planned, worked to our advantage by taking some of the sting out of parting. But now as I looked around the room, my cold resolve melted away, and I wanted nothing more than to continue teaching for another twenty weeks.

Anna Steinberg, a big woman with a heavy Russian accent under a raspy, cracking voice; Anna, who just turned ninety, is the first to greet me. She tentatively shoves a book across the table to where I'm sitting.

"Here, this is for you. My grandson gave it to me, but I wouldn't read it now, it's too big, too many pages, I just don't have the time. I thought you might like it." She waits a second while I leaf through, noting that her grandson had inscribed it.

"Well, does it interest you?"

I'm still stunned, but I manage a "Yes, it's great." The book is *The Brethren*, about the Supreme Court. One of the themes the group had worked on was justice. Almost all of Anna's stories revolved around some aspect of this theme. Her favorite goes something like this:

"When I was a little girl, maybe four-five years old, this is in Russia, we had a neighbor who had a beautiful little baby, that baby I went to play with every day. I loved that baby very much, maybe because it made me feel like a big girl. One day, as I was going out of the house to see the baby, my mother told me, 'You can't go there today, you can't go there any more to see the baby.' 'Why?' I said, and she told me that the baby died. I ran out of the house and went and saw the baby, dead, and I remember walking out of their home. I was on the street, crying, I looked up into the sky and said, 'You can't fool me, oh no, there is no such thing as a god who would take that poor innocent baby's life, there is no God who knows right from wrong'."

Anna has been the catalytic force of the workshop. She's been a Marxist since the days when she worked in the garment district, but her role as catalyst has less to do with her politics than with her personality. She tends to dominate the class by talking for great lengths of time. The other three women have openly rebelled against her, and Susan and I have spent a lot of our planning time trying to figure out a way to help her learn to edit her speeches. She is always asking for reassurance about herself as a person and needs the group, especially me, its leader, to tell her that we want her there.

Anna didn't do very much actual writing during the course of the workshop. In fact only one of the four women, Esther Taggert, wrote consistently. Esther is in her mid-seventies and healthy. She is one of the active members of the home, organizing the others, and generous with her time. She is a former teacher and preserves the rigor of that profession in her manner. Esther is very good at mediating disputes and steering a middle path between two antagonists. She usually writes short reportorial pieces that close with a subtle moral twist.

Ray Schwartz is the quiet one in the group; she began the workshop with a lot of spirit, but a cataract operation left her very weak and disoriented. It's quite a struggle for her, but she has managed to attend most of the sessions as a listener.

Helen Prinz, the fourth member, is blind; she is a small, frail woman who worked her whole life as a nurse. She is the opposite of Anna. A sharp dry wit, Helen is always making little jokes and is very critical of the other members of the group, particularly Anna. A typical scenario would have Anna talking for a long time, Helen finally becoming impatient and making a critical remark, Anna "taking it personally," and Esther jumping in to mediate the squabble. It got so rough at times that Anna would get up to leave. Once, in fact, she didn't come to class because of the difficulties she was having.

One day, after I was feeling particularly frustrated about the lack of writing being produced, Helen took me back to her room and handed me a sheaf of papers. In it were a dozen short stories, reminiscences, and essays. The work was excellent; her writing was perceptive and moving.

"I did write when I was able, you see, it's very hard now."

Susan comes into the lounge carrying a pot of fresh coffee, and I break open the box of pastries. Two apricot, two *mohn* (poppy seeds), and two prune. The tape recorder is turned on. Between bites of pastry and sips of coffee, I try to find out what the workshop has meant to everyone.

"For me, it was a good way to keep in touch with the outside world," Esther says.

"The discussions were stimulating and challenging," Helen says, "which is important in a place like this. It's easy to get lost playing bingo."

"It was a place for us to express ourselves," says Ray.

"It gives you a taste that you're somebody too," says Anna. She adds that for her the workshop was an important social activity; it gave her a chance to interact with people in a way she didn't normally do.

Susan, in private, later says that the workshop has been one of the best medications for the bruised egos that we see struggling along in these halls.

And what about me? They want to know what I felt about the workshop. Did I feel it was a success or failure? Were they good enough? Did I accomplish what I set out to do?

Suddenly, I'm nervous again; we're at a point where everything I say is crucial. I have a purpose in mind. I want to get them to do something that I'm not at all sure is possible. I want them to continue the workshop independently after I leave. I'm not sure why I want this; perhaps it is a feeling of guilt that motivates me. Guilt of many sorts. The guilt that comes from being powerless in a situation, yet somehow responsible for it—a sort of general malaise that afflicts those of us who have not yet adjusted to postmodern ex-

istence. Or perhaps it is the guilt of relief. The relief I felt whenever
I left the home. Not being the one who had to stay on, but being the
strong one, the young one, the healthy one. Or perhaps it was the
guilt I felt at not being able to confront my own personal horror of
growing old and feeble and helpless. I worked in a prison once,
Riker's Island men's house of detention, and every time I left the
island I would experience these feelings of guilt also. But they
weren't as strong or as personal. I didn't identify with the prisoners;
and though I felt in the main that it was society that sorely needed
reform and perhaps even detention, my feelings never went much
deeper than sociopolitical rage. But at the home I immediately see
my complicity in the crime. A token crumb of "culture" is being
tossed in at the last moment, not an attempt to alter the condition but
rather to make it a little less painful for the onlookers.

As I scan the faces of the people in the room—Helen, Esther, Anna, Ray, and Susan—I realize that guilt is not the whole explanation.
There is something good, quite good, that has happened for us during these weeks: it is simply that these women were allowed to
regain some of their lost dignity. They were given a chance to push
to a limit and allowed to fail or succeed. Such an option is often
missing in the homes, no matter how well-equipped or pleasant they
may be. One is really allowed to *do* only one thing once one enters:
die. Even this final act loses any possible grace and dignity in the
waiting-room atmosphere that enshrouds the residents.

So what we have done is somehow fight off death for a while; a
spirit emerged from the workshop. This "rage against the dying of
the light" is what I don't want to evaporate when I leave. This is
what I want to demand of my workshop participants: their struggle
must continue because it is only in the act of struggling that they will
be able to find a bit of peace and contentment. And it is my own
death, too, that I'm challenging here at the close of the workshop,
and that is even more frightening to me as I scan their faces. When I
walk out of the classroom, it's over, finished, kaput, that's it, no
more; and as with approaching death, one has to resolve and accept
all past regrets, all wishes and hopes. My way of dealing with those
wishes is not to resolve and accept, but to have the workshop continue.

But how can I, a kid, tell a ninety-year-old woman about facing
death? So I say instead, "I think it would be a great idea if the
workshop continued even though I'm going to have to leave. After
all, it's just a beginning that we have here, and now that you have a

good foundation and know each other, you don't really need me in order to continue getting something out of these meetings.'' They agree, although somewhat reluctantly. I'm told that it really won't be the same for them—and how important my presence is, and how much it means to them to have someone from ''the outside'' come and share their work. But I won't hear any of it. ''It's important for you to continue,'' I repeat. ''You can't stop now.'' There is an urgency in my voice. I believe what I'm saying. I believe they can do it. But as I look over to Susan for encouragement, I detect her veteran's sense of the futility of my urgings. It's almost enough to make me stop, but I still have enough steam left to get them to promise me that they will meet next week and to agree on a topic for their first independent discussion.

I'm pleased with myself on the subway ride home, so pleased that I barely notice that I'm on the cursed Lex. until the ride is almost over.

Three weeks later, I call Susan to find out how everything is going. The answer to my main question is: ''No.'' They met once but decided it was too hard for them to go it alone. Susan consoles me with the fact that new friendships and relationships, strong ones, have developed and that this is one of the most important things to come out of these workshops. Susan is probably right: one cannot expect miracles in such a short time; and if a couple of strong bonds developed, I should be pleased, and not forget that they wrote for a period of time, and that it meant something. But as for me, I have not yet learned how to accept happy endings.

Minerva's Doll

Janet Bloom

To give an impression of my writing workshop at Casita Maria Senior Center in Spanish Harlem, I have taken excerpts about one of our most deeply moving sequences from my weekly journal and inserted clarifications as needed. I noted then that I felt this part of the journal was being "written in the flickering of the flames."

This was the beginning of our second round of workshops. The first round had begun in April and concluded in August, 1979, with El Grupo Literario giving a glowing and warmly received reading of their work for the other members of the center. After a brief end-of-summer hiatus, everyone was glad and eager to be together again. We climbed up to our usual room on the second floor, in one of those standard, redbrick, cruciform project buildings, the halls of which often feel to me like a rainy day inside a submarine. So I am always glad to get to our light-filled corner room and see the long wooden table at the far end of which we sit. Except for the people, it is the only thing in the center of real substance, real grain, depth, color, and polish. It appears to have been well oiled, to bring out all the striations of reddish browns to yellows, then burnished like a dress shoe. It is our ground. We put our papers and elbows on it, and talk across it.

CASITA MARIA JOURNAL: 10/16/79 AND 10/23/79

This gathering seemed rather quiet, as we were working with a new interpreter. Except that Minerva Rios was bubbling with suggestions for our new start, which tickled me pink, and which I encouraged, as she has always treated me with the embarrassing respect she thinks proper to a teacher. To her especially, but also to the others—who never went beyond sixth grade in Puerto Rico, if they went to school at all—I am "la Maestra," the feminine for master, not in the sense of master craftsman, which I would like, but calling to mind a hickory-stick teacher with the right answer, the correct way. It is constant watchdog work to take any chance to step down from the position of authority they keep putting me (and how many others in their life?) into, and give them a leg up toward assuming the authority over themselves necessary to authorship.

I wanted us to be a little more orderly and studious than we had been and hoped now that we knew each other better, we might find a way of tailoring our work to common interests. My initial efforts to arrive at some agreement on a thematic organization for our work had drawn blanks from them, appeared to be utterly unreal to them, so I gave in and did whatever seemed appropriate moment by moment.

Now I wanted to try asserting more direction again. When I asked them to write down a list of what is most commonly *on their minds*, the complexity and abstraction of the things they listed were beyond the reach of any common focus that I could see, so I gave them an assignment, their first. I'm loath to give assignments in these circumstances as I think the benefit, the point of writing for people in groups like these, will come from their getting around to wanting to do it and cannot come from being told what to do. But now I felt selecting a focus might be useful, so I asked them to choose a very familiar and important object in their home and describe it. I emphasized once again that good writing comes out of familiarity.

The pickup on this assignment was astounding. Everyone delivered the following week. This had never happened before, when I'd made only suggestions as to what they write about. Minerva and Bernard Burgos, the two oldest members of the group, both in their seventies, delivered very moving pieces. Bernard had never written a word in all the previous twenty weeks and also had never said much, except once something about gambling.

When we discussed Juanita Rivera's and Alejandrina Diaz's pieces about their TV sets and what the different members liked on TV and why, Minerva said, "Because I am all alone. With TV I have company." She is a childless widow who used to work in a laundry and in restaurants. She graduated from elementary school in Puerto Rico and came over to this country in 1929, about the same time as Bernard. Most of the people in this center are living on less than $5,000 a year.

Juan Torres hadn't done the assignment, but had written instead about a recent visit to a Seattle winery on a trip to see his son. I was very pleased because, while not following my immediate directions, he was following an ongoing and deeper set of instructions. He was going on his own authority and writing about what was on his mind, which is all one can write about well since it is what one *cares* about at the moment.

Then came the *pièce de resistance*: Minerva's doll story. Someone called it "a living relic." As I do with much of both their prose and conversations, I have typed it out in lines as if it were poetry. Mechanically, this makes the back and forth between the Spanish and the English translation much easier going. More fundamentally, it transforms what feels in prose like an easy-to-lose scrap of life into a framed, full bodied, resonant, and somehow complete poetic moment. I want them to see the poetry in their lives. In a way I do not care if they ever write poems. Personal—otherwise known as creative—writing is a process which won't come easily or naturally to many. There is too much solitude and work in it for most people's taste, and then there's the problem of what you do with it after you've written it. But I do care that they *think* poems: people can use writing, or drawing, or talking as ways of learning how to see poetically, as ways of framing their experience in their minds so that they can turn it around and milk it for all it's worth, as a poet might. For me the following story, the written statement, was only the beginning of the poem we made when talking about the writing and living through something with Minerva.

El objeto mas querido que poseo

Escrita por Minerva Rios

De todos los objetos que poseo, en mi casa y que mas quiero,
es una vieja muñeca Española para adornar la cama.
Este muñeca me la trajeron de España hace mas de treinta anos.
Esta muneca tiene el cuerpo de trapo;
la cabeza es de un material como yeso
y los brazos como de plástico.
Ella era muy bonita. Digo "era"
porque ya su cabeza se está deteriorando.
Su cara está arreglada como una mujer.
Sus ejas, mejillas, uñas, y labios están pintados.

Tiene zapatos de taco alto.
Su cuerpo todavia está como nuevo.
¡Como recuerdo, a mi muñeca, vestida como una Española
con su traje de satén encajes negros
y su velo puesto por la cabeza hasta la cintura
y su elegante peineta,
adornando el centro de mi cama.
Ahora solo busco como podré reponerle la cabeza
o si se le podia rensovar la misma que tiene.

Minerva's own translation follows, with my more literal version of
some passages in parentheses.

The object that I own and I love
(The most loved object that I possess)

Of all the objects I own, in my house, and (that) I love (most),
is an old Spanish doll that adorns my bed.
This doll was brought to me from Spain more than thirty years ago.
This doll body is made of rags; (this doll has a body of rags)
but the head is made of clay; (is of a material like clay)
and the arms are like plastic.
She was very beautiful. I said "was"
because now the head is coming apart.
Her face is fixed like a real woman.
Her cheeks, eyebrows, nails and lips are painted.
She has high heels.
Her body is still like new.
Oh! how I remember my doll, dressed like a Spanish lady
sitting in the middle of my bed
with her elegant hair combed
and black lace veil down to her waist
and her satin and black lace dress.
She looked so beautiful adorning my bed.
Now I only look for a way by which I can find a new head
(look for how I could replace the head)
or fix the one she already has.
(the same that she has.)

More literally, the next to the last sentence reads:

(with her dress of black satin lace
and her veil placed from the head to the waist
and her elegant comb,
adorning the center of my bed.)

I asked everyone to say what the story meant. No one, except Juan, under his breath—he sits next to me because of his poor hearing—treated the story as directly symbolical of Minerva herself, now facing a cataract operation, and no doubt having faced for many years the very deep wrinkles of her face. Several said her story was about "conservation." One said it was about using the doll as a substitute daughter.

Minerva was in no way consciously connecting herself with the crumbling face of her doll.

I was fascinated and felt I had to be careful in guarding the secret and not being too direct about the meaning of the story. After learning everyone's reactions, I asked Minerva if she felt she could or wanted to expand on her story. She wanted to know if I thought she should. I said I thought it was very beautiful the way it was, but I also thought she knew more about the doll and could tell more if she wanted to. It was up to her; I didn't want to pressure her. I think she liked the idea of trying to see if there was more. She wanted me to tell her what. I said I couldn't do that, but she'd heard what the story meant to others, and maybe she could answer those things a little.

Then we went on to Bernard's partly written, partly told story of young love thwarted by parents who interfered with it on race and class grounds. The important object in his house, a photograph of a tambourine player which he has hung surrounded with musical instruments, reminded him of a dance where this twist in his fate began.

CASITA MARIA JOURNAL: 10/30/79 AND 11/6/79

Breathless. Hair-raising.

Once you have a choice of saying something or not, what an edge you're on! And if it's about love! Or death!

In the shower this morning, getting ready to go to Casita Maria, I came to a new understanding of understanding. Quite suddenly I caught on to something new in what a friend had said to me months before. It seemed as if I had only caught and been tossing around the outside of the ball before. Now I'd caught the inside. And my future seemed to depend on how I fielded that new catch. Then it occurred to me that Minerva's life also depends on how I field the inside of her story while others were fielding only the outside of it.

So I was full of speculation about whether or not, or when, to reveal what I'd caught. Ever since we'd read the story, I'd kept trying to figure out what I might say to her or ask her about the relation between her operation and her doll. As we settled down around the table, Alejandrina said Minerva had brought her doll. In a few minutes, sure enough! Minerva buzzes in with a doll that seems bigger than she. It was quite different from my expectation. She was a lived-in doll, and I had had a stage doll or a store doll in mind. The doll was really only a medium-sized doll, a foot and a half to two feet tall, but she seemed very large when Minerva sat her down in the middle of the table and spread out full circle all the layers of her black-lace-trimmed, red taffeta, ruffled skirt. There had been no mention of red taffeta with the black satin and lace in the story. I have no recollection of her torso. She had naked arms, very shapely, Capezio feet, and a very poignant face. The others focused on the peeled and cracking paint on the face. But more powerful to me was the effect of the shadow over the eyes, in the manner of the current dark fashion in eyeshadowing. She was like a pubescent doll painted by Goya. There was sorrow and dignity in her face that has never gotten within miles of an American doll I've ever seen. Her rosebud lips evoked in me a whole pantomime of the containment of manners: prissy is too strong a word for this; everything seemed shaped and patted together (perhaps because of Minerva's pats in displaying her) so as not to run wild or leak. And what Bernard noticed, and put so well—I don't have his exact words: a faraway look, a look as if she were thinking of someone not there. We worked on describing that expression at the very end of the session.

Minerva, in her brisk way, plunked the doll down, then showed us her feet, spread out her skirts, pointed to the arms and pinched them, and kept knocking on the arm nearest her and on the head. Her concern, her insistent concern throughout, was the "material" of the body. She kept wondering why the arms were all right while the face was cracking. Minerva is a very active person, more wiry than bouncy, not sedentary or contemplative, but executive; she's the president of the women's club at the center, and a showwoman. She loves to recite poetry at parties, which is not uncommon at Puerto Rican festivities. Finished with all the gesturing involved in her guided tour of her doll, she lay the doll down. I could hardly bear it, the doll lying out there, feet to us, just a little of the profile we were talking about visible at the far end of the table. I asked Minerva to sit her up, prop her up against her purse. Minerva was slow in understanding what I wanted; it seemed so obvious. When she finally tried to sit her up, the doll wanted to slip forward feet first, and Bernard helped push her back.

He told us his wife has a doll like this, but she is black. He quietly proclaimed this with a twinkly look over to me. He's very light. Never having thought of him as black until the subject came up in his story of young love, I now sensed it was a very deep concern and wondered if his wife has a darker complexion than he. I haven't found a way yet to get more deeply into this. I know only that it seems in Puerto Rico people can be proud of some aspects of their mixed racial heritage, but here they are confounded with a prejudice so deep I was unable to make the group enrollment mixed. Mysteriously the interested blacks in this largely Puerto Rican center never came.

I soon got the idea of asking everyone to write about the face of the doll and the meaning of what was happening to it, and passed out paper. Meanwhile the question of the material the doll is made of was disputed at length. Her arm did feel like plastic, but that seemed impossible for a thirty-year-old Spanish doll. Bernard, formerly a housepainter, gave a word in Spanish which turned out to mean plaster. Maybe. Definitely not china. I suggested to Minerva that whatever the material was, it seemed as if the skin color were "baked" into it, but the features of the face were painted over that. She kept saying in many ways that she wanted to get it fixed. Did I know how? I said I'd seen a doll hospital near Bloomingdale's that I had long wanted to take my doll to. Much later I finally dared to say that I thought it would be very expensive. She told Damaris, the interpreter, she'd pay $50. My view of the material satisfied Minerva to the extent that she knocked on the head and said, "It's good inside." Did I support that idea enough? Before I left the center I meant to go through the yellow pages with her, looking for doll hospitals. (I'll call her in a little while, and we'll do it over the phone.)

When the writing about the face started, Minerva wanted some prompting from me. I said I didn't want to steer; I wanted them to find their way. But it occurred to me that one word from the others, giving a clue to their point of view, might jiggle something loose for her. So I asked them each to give us one word for the face. Juan obliged immediately with "aging." Alejandrina inevitably started to make a speech. I insisted she stop. So did Damaris. Finally Alejandrina got it down to "painting." Bernard didn't get it down to one word either. Minerva's word was "material." Her request for some prompting set me off on an important speech.

In the last few weeks of teaching in public school I've been concerned with teaching stream of consciousness and how to enter the imagination to my fifth grade class. I said: Minerva's question seems to say that I know what she should write. I don't. I told them about the way a painter friend of mine taught painting: by having the whole class write down descriptions, verbal sketches really, of the paintings up before us for discussion. I suggested they start out just describing the face, and in the description they would find the clues that would lead them into the solution of the mystery of what they were going to write about the meaning of the face. I really love this formulation for helping people get over the terrible blank about what to write. Why do we expect ourselves to know so much, to know the answer before we've even found the question, when, if we devoted our whole lives to it, we'd still know so little? Minerva smiled, happy with what I'd said. Bernard and Juan were also happy with it, nodding in assent several times. These smiles meant a lot to me. They seemed to be the smiles of getting into the excitement. Each one had the happiness of a child let into a ring of hands.

Here's what they wrote, in the order in which we read it aloud for discussion. Minerva took hers with her. (I've asked for it repeatedly, and she promises to look for it, but can't until she gets her new glasses and can really see again.)

Minerva's Doll

La muñeca parece que un tiempo
era una preciosa y hermosa doncella.
Hoy después de los años que le han pasado
en el rostro las huellas han dejado.

The doll appears as if once
she was a very precious and beautiful lady.
Today after the years she has gone through
the marks are left on her face.—Juan Torres

Esta muñeca de Minerva es una flape;

es una muñeca muy vieja de tanto años.
Pero para tener tanto años se ve bien.

Tiene un poco la cara escrachada
pero ella puede pintarla con una pintura
que se llama vasnil y queda perfecta.

Yo me siento muy contenta por ver
una muñeca de tantos anos.

Minerva's doll is a flapper;
it is a very old doll of many years.
But having so many years she looks good.

Her face is a little scratched
but she can paint it with paint
called varnish and it will be perfect.

I feel very happy to see
a doll of so many years—Alejandrina Diaz

La cara de esta muñeca a mi entender
fue pintada. Y con las años le esta pasando
como nos pasa a nosotros las personas humana,
que la cara cambia.

Yo me refiero a la cara es que
le pasa igual que la cara de una persona cuando es joven,
y cuando llega a la hedad madura
la cara cambia, las arrugas y also mas.

The face of this doll to my understanding
was painted. And with the years it's happening
as it happens to us human beings,
that the face changes.

I am referring to the face: what
happened to it is the same as what happens to the face
of a person when young,
and when he reaches the age of maturity
the face changes, the wrinkles and something more.—Bernard
  Burgos

I am sorry that Juanita's reactions were not recorded. Never having been to school, she does not write; but she is our natural poet. All her life she has composed poems and songs and loves to slip a song into our sessions in her bell-clear voice. The interpreters or I have taken some of her work down, but this time we missed.

At some point in the rush of reactions, I went around trying to help them distinguish and elaborate on their separate points of view. Bernard's remains clear. He seemed to feel that one has a whole new face. Minerva's view was that the material underneath is as good as new. I teased Juan a good deal, on the basis of a misunderstanding from both handwriting and translation, that he wasn't telling what his point of view was; that, as far as I could make out, it was perfectly ambiguous: he could mean either that age left many marks, or that, given the age, there were few marks. He stubbornly wanted to leave it at the "objective" statement: age leaves marks. Then he seemed to come out in favor of the second view, which led me into Alejandrina's having said the face was "a little scratched." I am sorry I did not pick up on the acceptance in her last sentence, but I was eager to tell a story, especially as she was insisting on the varnish.

I had already said this doll's face was painted by someone as skillful as a portrait painter. Now I told them that I had been in love with a painter whose words I respected very much. And when I came home from Paris with a bronze candlestick which was heavily tarnished deep brown, I told him I was going to polish it. I could not have been more shocked by the lecture he gave me. He really read me out, saying I should take it as it came, with the patina of its life history. I told them that I can still be as ashamed as I was then, whenever I find myself wanting to polish the life off of something, when I see myself wanting to clean something up that is better accepted with respect for its age and history. I added that this is a very profound question, which keeps coming up over and over again in life. There was a lot of nodding.

More and more things came out about Minerva's doll. She said her living room is not very fixed up, but her bedroom gets a lot of attention. I'd missed this, but it had made an impression on Damaris, who is studying home economics. Later it occurred to me what a wonderful story could be made about the woman who fixes up her bedroom, "her interior," as Damaris put it, not her front room.

Minerva told us how she didn't have this doll on her bed all the time. She has lots of dolls, including the ones she has made. (Doll making is popular among Puerto Rican women. This center has classes in it, and the bazaars held to raise money for center expenses are always filled with them. Minerva made me one for Christmas, and she gave it to me with a card attached to the bonnet tie saying: "To my dear teacher. . .; Para mi querida maestra. . ." These dolls are all bright, pretty, elegant lady dolls). She said she takes this Spanish doll out of its box only on two holidays when she is having visitors. One is New Years; I'm not quite sure of the other. She puts a comb in her hair and a black veil over her. I'm not sure if the veil is to cover her lack of hair—Minerva also wants to get her a wig—or for a tradition, or both. This skirt was made, I guess not by Minerva, to replace the original which got old, dirty, worn out. It was in telling us about the special occasions on which she brought out this doll that she said, "There's a superstition that it's unlucky to have a doll on your bed." To this Bernard immediately added the one about it being unlucky to have a hat on your bed.

My first thought was of the resemblance between a doll and a corpse. Then I thought of the sainted Mother Cabrini laid out in her habit up near the Cloisters, and those medieval couples with their dog, faithful as a stone rose, lying in European churches. I felt I understood immediately that the superstition about having a doll on your bed arose from the resemblance between a doll and a dead person. And I understood the hat one similarly, as having to do with a missing person. I asked them what they thought the superstitions were about. No one was saying. They really had no tracks to run on. I left the question hanging as long as I could, angling it differently, but nothing was forthcoming, so I landed my thought on them. Juan tugged at me and offered to get me lunch. I could have wrung his neck. I put him by. It was time for lunch, but now, after seven months of working together, we had for the first time raised the subject of death.

It had come up once when Juan had told us of the time when he put a gun to his head after a youthful failure in love, but the coldness of the gun stopped him from pulling the trigger. That day several others told stories of suicide and love, but not personal stories like Juan's, and all those stories were of long ago and far away. Today, for the first time, we all knew that one of the group members was going to the hospital for an operation. The moment went very swiftly. I'd said it. Should I have?

Up to this point, Minerva had kept insisting that the material the doll's head is made of is good and that the trouble was only the paint. I had supported her in that and was really tickled with her pluck. Now she began telling us about her sister who won't go into an elevator, but she, herself, goes into an elevator figuring, if it breaks, they fix it! She said her sister's worry made bad things happen, and I agreed, saying it sounded as if her sister drew the trouble out. Then it occurred to me to say to Minerva that her attitude made things go as well as possible. She dismissed this suggestion. The way she had put it initially made it seem as if she saw herself going around not knowing what's happening so that anything bad just hits her on the head. I wanted her to know that my very firm feeling about her is that she knows what is happening; she just doesn't worry about it, and she makes the best of it by thinking that if anything goes wrong they will fix it.

Afterward, Damaris surprised me, when I asked her about it, by saying that she thought I shouldn't have mentioned a doll's resemblance to a corpse. She was sure that was why Juan offered me lunch. I said, "But didn't Minerva then give herself a big pep talk? And, if that's so, then didn't mentioning death help Minerva make herself feel stronger?" Thinking about that, Damaris decided what I had done wasn't all bad. But she maintained that Minerva's pride was in for a downfall, that everybody was used to her being strong, and that it left her very vulnerable with nobody, including herself, recognizing her fear. Damaris thought Minerva would suffer worse if things came out badly. I said, "But it's the same act that's going to help her pull the pieces together then. I am putting my faith in the act." But, at the same time, by asking the others to give her their views, I was also trying to provide her with a sense that there were ways other than her own of accommodating the situation, ways she could reach out for so that she would not be at a total loss if her way, her faith in fixing, was not borne out. I wanted to begin opening all of them to the availability of other viewpoints on a subject which had been totally locked up—viewpoints which they might use to ease their minds of some of the terrible pressures they are all under about the repairability and decay of their bodies.

I loved Minerva's pep talk. However Damaris made me wonder if my feeling that Minerva is in good shape and good spirits for her operation is just a case of opposites attract. Perhaps I, who usually think they might not fix it, may simply be enjoying the relief of the opposite viewpoint, though it seems clear to me that Minerva is no dope and knows as well as anyone what the hazards and worst possibilities are.

By misfortune or good fortune all this had gone on while I was thinking that Minerva's operation was still a few weeks off. Very near the end of this class I was told she was going into the hospital next Sunday. When we broke up for lunch, I thanked her for bringing in the doll, and she said, very emphatically, she had wanted *me* to see it before she went into the hospital. The way she said it, I felt as if she were giving me her soul, as if she had said, ''I'm going, you keep me.'' Whatever it was, I *had* to have it, a legacy pressed hard into my hand.

Such momentous things happen without one's knowing. Afterward I saw that she, the one in danger, had thrown her lifeline to me on shore. At that moment she was letting me know. Suddenly, across that table, we had a life-and-death bond, as deep as bonds between close relatives, so deep that both people wear blinders, or speak without mentioning the true subject, in order to see their way through the moment. A minute before that we didn't have it. I see it now as a reverse umbilical cord, being attached at the end, rather than cut off at the beginning of life.

Again I was astonished. But now I felt in no way prepared for the burden, or the joy of the burden of this trust. Later I recalled the women in the Artists & Elders Astoria Workshop whom I'd interviewed! They felt the other people in their group were friends even more than the people they had called friends throughout their lives. What had happened with Minerva seemed something like that, an incredible leap of trust in a stranger, a bridging, which suddenly enables a person to give to the outside world something it has made her keep terribly private all those years; a burden so heavy and so explosive a person can't dare to reveal it to those she is closely bound to; a terrible giving, terrible only because it comes so late, but wonderful and softening too. I hear Irene Salamon's voice speaking of this in the Astoria Workshop. It was so relaxing for her to testify about this unimaginable friendship that had come to her. I cried then; I'm crying now. I see Minerva's very deeply weathered face, usually taut, active, pert, let down a little after she pressed that giving into me. She was relaxed, a little drained, and softened by some deep recognition and acceptance of a legacy delivered. Perhaps all of us want to leave a legacy with someone in the world outside the family. A childless widow has no one else to turn to. It was as if she had asked me to see her, recognize her in one of the most feared moments. And that glimpse I gave her was somehow a relief.

When Minerva and Bernard delivered up their stories, I sensed they felt something newborn in themselves. It seemed to me they were more deeply happy and excited about this feeling because they are closer to death and have little time to live with it—the giving and the taking away, an exhilarating somersault at any age, but increasingly exquisite.

As Minerva told us she had lots of dolls, I said then I bet you have lots of stories. When I found her to say goodbye as I was leaving the center for the day, she and Bernard, who is president of the men's club, were working over the bingo accounts. All I could think to say, as a way of going with her in spirit to the hospital, was to put it in her head to think about what she would write while there. She said with a girlish secrecy, "Did you know people used to talk with fans? You know, when boys and girls couldn't talk to each other because their parents were watching, they could do this with the fan," and she touched her fingers to her lips, indicating a kiss in fan talk. Her sensuality seemed to be flaring in her imagination before possible blindness, before death.

When the group went to visit her in the hospital the following week, she was sitting up in the middle of her bed with her legs crossed, almost as pert as ever. None of the usual color of makeup was on her face; the always neat hair was a little mussed; she had a big white eye patch and a bright pink quilted bedjacket. She didn't even want me to roll the back of her bed up. I thought: isn't that just like her. Finally, though, she let me. And when she had relaxed into the backrest a little, she said how much she loved the way we talked of *recuerdos del ayer*, memories of yesterday, and she mentioned Juan's story of the coldness of the gun.

A woman came into the room dressed in nurse's whites, and Minerva introduced her as the sister with whom she'd be staying after the hospital. Several weeks later I found out quite accidentally that this sister had in fact not taken her in and she'd had to go from friend to friend until she could take care of herself alone. She had friends, this time. But I am under the impression that many of the old people have difficulty making friends precisely because they are so much at the mercy of failing health and failing means to help themselves or others. For some, their memories of yesterday are their only friends, the only things they have to see them through. Minerva's thankfulness for our talk and her experience on getting out of the hospital make me see the work of these groups is to provide sustenance and light for people who live in the very dark perspective of the likely eclipse of friendship and help.

Could I have done more for Minerva if I'd known the exact date of her operation? I would have done something else no doubt. Could it have fallen out so well? In a way the whole story is a story of getting *more* meaning out of *not* knowing as we usually expect ourselves to know.

Did more get said through the indirectness I harbored by not insisting on identifying the X in the symbolic equation of Minerva and the doll? I think so. There is something terrible—perhaps owing to widespread therapy—about the way we label and box and point at things, as if we could pin them down or dismiss them, as if they have no mystery. By not discussing the doll as symbolizing Minerva's concerns about her operation, blindness, and death, which would have restricted the conversation to things about which we are all more or less helpless, the discussion was open to everything from attitudes toward elevator repair to fan kisses. Staying with the symbol seemed like opening a window in an airless room, or like staying in the garden of life, instead of going over to the chalk on the blackboard and nailing down meaning with squeaking chalk the way we nail corpses into coffins, as if meaning would not get out alive. We all know better; for instance, we get the meaning of incredibly complex and fluid facial movements all the time. Perhaps the terror of discussing death is simply a terror of having nothing to say about it. It hasn't happened yet. We haven't met any returning travelers. Once beyond the impossibility of feeling obliged to say something about something one can know nothing about, there's plenty to say. It might be said that by withholding the interpretation of Minerva's doll story, which could have been death to our conversation, I enabled us to circumnavigate the void, feel out ways of approaching it. Because we were only dimly cognizant of what the doll was meaning, it acquired full meaning, true meaning; it swam in the sea of our thought.

Even Alejandrina became engrossed in something outside herself.

I want to convey something of this very odd sense of responsibility I have just come into. Responsibility for the mystery? I'm not sure exactly. If somebody can say something so moving to you that you cannot move, something the dawning of which is so important, so profound, that you could not let yourself know in words what it meant when it was said to you, but had to wait an hour or more until, in a protected solitary moment in a dark stairwell, it dawned on you; if the meaning of something important can take months or years to come through to you, then, in what tense do you deal with meaning as a teacher? Do you aim for meaning now, or meaning later?

Maybe I am only going over a personal ridge. Someone asked me many years ago: "Do you have to be so pointy?" That's been going off in me like the grains of a time capsule ever since. He meant: did I always have to point out the meaning of everything? I began to see that pointing can make a subject squirm, pin it down in a damaging way, jab the life out of it, make it go away. A softer response seems better sometimes, more attractive, more welcoming. By now I feel that neither approach alone is the answer to how best to listen to people. At one moment the softer approach may draw more into view. At another moment in the same situation, a thrust may open more up. It's a matter of trusting your intuition, your touch, at any given moment. This trust is developed, I guess, through the practice one gets in friendships, trying out harder and softer approaches and seeing which is most effective when, and with whom. You develop an ear for those moments when a person can live and live more within a symbol—when thoughts will flourish by remaining inside the cave of the symbol, protected from interpretation, as dreams are while they're growing, for instance—and an ear for the other sort of moments when thoughts will flourish from the direction given to them by interpretation. It's a choice between swimming around and walking, or between flying around and running straight to the point. It's a choice between dwelling in the garden of the imagination or following the geometric roadways of the intellect; between receiving, accepting, or analyzing critically. These are two very opposing impulses which can be contained in different moments of the same situation, as with Minerva's doll.

Now that I can point if I want or have to, I was fearless enough in the workshop to float in the black pulse of the mystery and let it push me to mention corpses. The fearlessness may simply be a highly practiced and therefore calloused fearfulness. In any case, I sense myself to be peculiarly unafraid of the subject of death and therefore quite sensitive to other people's fears of discussing it.

I am all questions and amazement tonight. Having spent years as a writer devoted to self-scrutiny and to the scrutiny of life, what can I aim to get across to people for whom life mostly just happens? When you think about it, how much do we learn in school, at home, at church, about the thought processes of being human? It isn't learned from books. I think most of us know most of what we know about being human by accident, by what falls between the cracks, by getting burned. Someone very accidentally says something that means something to you, and you remember it the rest of your life; it comes back to you repeatedly, like lightning. I remember that candlestick story I told them today with hot flashes; I remember it by shame. We go around thinking we're supposed to remember the neutral or neutralized information they try to teach us in school; but actually we remember by shame, and happiness, and sorrow. The by heart part. The language has it right, even when we can't hear it any longer. We remember by heart, by what gets branded on our hearts. I am teaching branding irons. Today I am in awe of teaching branding irons. When these workshops begin to work for all they are worth, what people begin to reveal is the brands they've had to cover up all their lives, literal brands in the case of concentration camp refugees, name brands in racist and other categorizing, imprisoning situations. And giving others a little glimpse of the terror is somehow an immense relief.

Teaching branding irons: it is like telling Minerva, after she has taken pains to tell us that she brings the doll out only on special occasions, that the superstition about a doll on your bed being unlucky is based on a doll's resemblance to a corpse. It's like laying a black egg.

The truth helps me, which makes me feel peculiar when I see it means trouble to others. There was a man who used to tell me the truth; he was in a way the first who did. I loved him for it. It made me feel more secure, anchored even, no matter how rough or shocking or breathtaking it was on impact. But he loved me. And since he died, I have taken the truth well from others because I can remember the love surrounding his harsh knowledge. So who am I to go into a senior center, which is sort of like a country club where people's pretenses are important, and tell the truth? As my mother would say, "It makes my gizzard wobble." The whole truth and nothing but the truth. Where did we ever get the idea of mouthing such a statement? As T. S. Eliot put it, "Humankind can't bear very much reality."

What is it they don't want to know? That they are going to die? Who doesn't know that? Is it possible that there is wisdom in their not wanting to know? In not wanting to go around thinking "they won't fix it this time." Is the wisdom of it simply that it's more fun not pinning things down or more fun pinning the tail on the donkey in all the wrong places because it goes there too?

Meaning. Something is going off in me about meaning. As if nobody ever told me about meaning, never even hinted at what it was all about. I started our group today talking about what meaning was all about, and how, if you paid the utmost attention, you

couldn't begin to catch up with it, so we couldn't get very close with
a lot of distractions. How can it be that our education has tried to
make it all stand still and be simple? How can that be? I simply do
not understand. The continents have always been surrounded by
oceans; we have always breathed air; they all flow. I don't understand. A word is a name, is a label pinned on like a paper tail. Meanwhile nothing stands still. And a word, like snow, is always becoming something else. And we can't talk about death, because we
spell it, say it with a capital D, and make it stare us in the face as if it
stood still. In my experience a dead lover never stands still; thoughts
of him run through my mind in new combinations and contexts
almost as if he were alive. He's not fixed. My perspective on him
changes. O.K., I am devoted to changing my mind. I had to be. But
even so, I never met a mind like a tombstone.

Right after he died people would say something to me about my
grief. I always wanted to say: What is it? They seemed to know, to
have some identifiable, isolatable phenomena in mind. I never
asked, perhaps knowing they wouldn't like the question, as well as
knowing I'd find out for myself, make my own grief. Almost ten
years later I met a very white-haired composer at an artist's colony.
She was in her sixties or seventies, I suppose, and recently wid-
owed. She was very reserved, and I don't know what it was about
me that broke that reserve enough for her to tell me that all her
friends kept telling her she'd get over it. "Get over it?" I said, hor-
rified. "You don't get over it. You live with it." She was so relieved. She thought there was something terribly wrong with her
that her grief for her husband, to whom she'd been married for over
thirty years, didn't go away the way people said it would. She seemed to have been told to sweep a lifetime of memories under the
carpet, and somehow my remarks gave them back to her. We
dismiss an awful lot. When we think we are dismissing pain, we are
in fact dismissing essential nourishment.

Whatever this composer saw in me must be akin to what Minerva
saw, enabling her to give me what I call her soul, her emotional
legacy. What is it? Is it simply that they both somehow felt if they
gave me a glimpse of the death they were grappling with, I could
take it, receive it? Not rebuff it or them? I think I am coming close
to the truth here. Compared with many if not most people I meet,
who seem to have death hanging from a pair of very lengthy tongs,
or have death invisibly biting their tail, I am not squeamish about it
mentally. I've lived very close to it for many years, as many people

have, more than we know. The reading and writing of poetry, which so often dwells on transiencies, has put me at ease with and given me a grip on the many guises of death. This does not mean that I don't get scared in subways or on street corners when a big truck or evil-looking man is coming at me. But whatever fright I experience is mostly contained; I recognize it, what it's about. Sometimes I take it as the lightning striking the darkness under the hood which sparks my propulsion system. And sometimes I think my fear is funny; I mean it is comic the way it comes barreling at me almost out of nowhere.

Through the experience of Minerva's doll, I am sensing that what I can do as a poet, for older people particularly, is give them their death, something society persists in trying to take away from people, by treating death as if the only thing to do with it is get over it, jump it, or get it over with as fast as possible. That, of course, makes it difficult to think or talk about death or the approach to death and impossible to learn that we all know how to live with death, our own and others! We live—all of us, all our lives—in more or less conscious fear of or desire for death, with people and things we are fond of coming and going, being given and taken away. We all have a lot of experience with and therefore accumulated strengths for handling transiencies, disappearances, hostilities, and humiliations of all sorts. We nearly die of laughter, shame, embarrassment, joy. But then most people leave any elaborations about these conjunctions to the poets, playwrights, and novelists, and go about thinking of death as black, of death as if it were only the obituary or the tombstone. In fact it is with us like water, like air; it is part of the daily flow and traffic of life. By ignoring it, treating it as unmentionable, we let it seep uncontrollably into our lives in forms as diverse as war and pollution.

If we could come to see death not as a big new subject, totally unknown, unknowable and terrifying, but as a daily experience which makes more or less frontal appearances in small disappointments as well as in funerals, then we need only tap strengths we already know we have to face physical death, whether or not we believe it's final.

II. CONCEPTS AND PRACTICES

The Uses of Reminiscence:
A Discussion of the Formative Literature

Marc Kaminsky

1. IMAGES OF REMINISCENCE

From ancient times, reminiscence has been particularly associated with old age, and attitudes towards remembering the past have long been a measure of a society's attitude towards its old people. In preliterate societies, elders often occupied positions of power and dignity because it was upon their memories that the transmission of culture depended. In present-day societies, however, many kinds of knowledge quickly become obsolete; books are a more reliable warehouse of the accumulated wisdom of the past; and memory is no longer an invaluable social asset. The position of old people has paralleled the declining fortunes of reminiscence: it is no longer held in high esteem as a storehouse of cultural riches, and neither are they. What makes the recent reevaluation of reminiscence so culturally significant is that nothing less than our attitude towards old people is at stake.

One of the more persistent images of old age fuses, or rather confuses, the age-old activity or reminiscence with hopelessness, denial of death, turning away from present realities, loss of memory, and intellectual deterioration. In the *Rhetoric*, Aristotle wrote of old people that "They live by memory rather than by hope, for what is left to them of life is but little compared to the long past. This, again, is the cause of their loquacity. They are continually talking of the past, because they enjoy remembering.[1] This passage is less remarkable in its error than in its perspicacity. The conviction that old age is necessarily hopeless because of its close proximity to death is still with us, and still distorts our perception of old people. Of great interest is Aristotle's recognition of the value of reminiscence: it is not only a source of pleasure, but it helps old people cope with their knowledge of the imminence of death.

137

It is startling to find Aristotle's view of the matter so closely echoed twenty-four centuries later in the gerontological literature. Take, for example, the following thumbnail sketch of "the aging process":

> In the psychological area, [the elderly person] may suffer from organic mental deterioration. His loss of memory may be marked and he may have a lessened capacity for grasping or understanding ideas. Moreover, the aging person is usually preoccupied with the past. While the younger person is inclined to look forward to "tomorrow" the older person's "tomorrow" may be the end of his life. It is for this reason that a preoccupation with the past can be a helpful defense in the older person's efforts to survive.[2]

This passage, which is representative of enlightened professional opinion of fifteen years ago, agrees with Aristotle in viewing denial of death as the chief motive for reminiscence. Furthermore, it loosely associates reminiscence with "organic mental deterioration." It does not seek to define precisely the relationship between "organic" impairment and a "preoccupation with the past," but freely allows us to assume that reminiscence is a somewhat pathological mental activity which is the result of senescent changes. A kind of half-conscious syllogism governs this view of reminiscence: since reminiscence is the characteristic activity of old age, and since old age is characterized by a general deterioration of intellectual and emotional capacities, then it must follow that reminiscence is a sign of senescent impairment. This stereotypical "portrait" of aging does not begin to suggest the clinically pejorative tone of the negative—and until quite recently, prevalent—view of reminiscence. Dr. Theodore Lidz, whose text is used to induct so many social work and medical students into knowledge of *The Person: His Development Throughout the Life Cycle*, offers us a compendium of demeaning "insights" veiled as neutrally causal explanations. Significantly enough, he discusses reminiscence under the chapter subtitle of "Memory Impairments":

> Elderly people, as is well known, spend an increasing amount of time talking and thinking about the past. It seems natural that as they feel out of the run of things, they should turn back to the days when life was more rewarding and enjoyable, and when events had a deeper impact on them. When the future

holds little, and thinking about it arouses thoughts of death, interest will turn regressively to earlier years. Still, in most persons who become very old, the defect is more profound. The person becomes unable to recall recent events and lives more and more in the remote past, as if a shade were being pulled down over recent happenings, until nothing remains except memories of childhood. This type of memory failure depends on senile changes in the brain and is perhaps the most characteristic feature of senility. We do not properly understand why earlier memories are retained while more recent happenings are lost.[3]

Dr. Lidz is hardly alone in viewing reminiscence as a "defect": the traditional and "common sense" view of our culture, of which Dr. Lidz is an authoritative representative, also equates reminiscence and regression, and sees it as the royal road to the proverbial "second childhood." As with sexuality, so with reminiscence: old people themselves adopt the conventional wisdom about themselves and become fearful of reminiscing:

> Our population [of old people] showed the effects of this common attitude. They hesitated to talk about the past because they did not want to be characterized as old people and because they did not want to meet with rejection. Consequently, they were conflicted about this and often criticized one another for being guilty of such behavior.[4]

The old people whom Aristotle described were at least better off in this respect: they still could "enjoy remembering" without the intervention of a cultural bias against the elderly which cloaked itself in the garb of psychosocial wisdom. They, like the horses to which Dr. Lidz metaphorically compares old people, may have been "out of the run of things," but they at least deemed reminiscence the natural, and even honorific, activity of old age.

2. LOSS OF MEMORY

The present state of our knowledge about memory function has been described as "equivocal."[5] There are, for example, studies which show that "the memory decline which accompanies aging seems to involve long-term memory forgetting rather than short-term memory.''[6] There are also ''A number of recent studies of memory function in the aged [that] have encountered great difficulty in explaining the apparently greater impairment of recent memory as compared with remote memory on organic grounds alone, and have suggested that emotional and motivational factors contribute significantly to this finding. There appears to be a complex inter-relationship of physical and emotional factors at work in senescence affecting both memory and learning.''[7] Then, too, there are studies which indicate that ''the decline with age in memory performance is attributable to the decline with age in learning performance.''[8] Hulicka and Weiss found that the old people whom they tested needed more time than younger people to learn new material; ''but once having learned the material, they retained equally when compared to the young.''[9] Finally, there are studies which ''require us to consider most of the intellectual decline in the healthy old to be a myth.''[10]

These studies, with their contradictory emphases and results, demonstrate that it is not easy to sift out the kernels of truth which lie scattered in the sands of our culture's prejudice against reminiscence. They are reviewed here for the sake of the coherent and affirmative view which they jointly make. Most of the evidence we have attests to ''the greater impairment of recent memory as compared with remote memory.'' The knotty problem which has yet to be unequivocally disentangled has to do with the factors which cause impairment of recent memory. Now, learning and memory are not functionally independent,[11] and a number of studies have found that there are ''no age differences in recall performance when acquisition [of new material] was equalized for young and old.''[12] Apparent memory impairment, then, would be caused by a ''deficit in cognitive ability'' in the old.[13] However, in challenging the ''myth of intellectual decline,'' several studies have shown

> with great clarity that a much larger proportion of the variance associated with age can be attributed to generation difference than to ontogenetic change. . . . In other words, there is strong evidence that much of the difference in performance on intellectual abilities between young and old is *not* due to decline in ability on the part of the old, but due to higher performance levels in successive generations.[14]

These studies demonstrate that the earlier cross sectional studies of intelligence confound individual development with sociocultural change, and do not take into account "motivational factors which may indeed interfere in the performance of old adults on intelligence tests as well as life tasks designed for the young."[15]

If impairment of recent memory is actually a sign of intellectual deterioration, and intellectual decline is in large measure a myth, how are we then to account for the memory loss that is commonly observed in old people? Is this, too, like the apparent decline in intellectual functioning, "at best a methodological artifact and at worst a popular misunderstanding?"[16] In summarizing the findings of a long-term study on normal aging conducted at the National Institute of Mental Health (NIMH), Dr. Robert Butler writes:

> To our surprise, we found that psychological flexibility, resourcefulness, and optimism, rather than the stereotype of rigidity, characterized the group we studied. Many of the manifestations heretofore attributed to aging per se clearly reflected medical illnesses, personality factors, and sociocultural effects. The belief that cerebral (brain) blood flow and oxygen consumption necessarily decreased as a result of chronological aging was not confirmed. It was found, rather, that when such changes occurred they probably resulted from vascular disease. The forty-seven men in our sample who were over sixty-five were found to have cerebral physiological and intellectual functions that compared favorably with a young control group. Intellectual abilities declined not as a consequence of the mysterious process of aging but rather as the result of specific diseases. Therefore, senility is not an inevitable outcome of aging.[17]

In the absence of organicity and specific diseases, we must examine "the motivational and emotional factors" which may be manifested as memory loss.

That memory loss may, in fact, be a manifestation of anxiety has been repeatedly confirmed in the literature on treatment of the elderly. We know that anxiety is the "constant companion" of old people, and that they have been "singled out to be its special prey."[18] Dr. Muriel Oberleder writes:

> It is true that certain symptoms appear more frequently in old age. However, I do not feel they are necessarily due to old age

any more than drug addiction is due to adolescence or bedwetting to childhood. A person usually chooses the symptom appropriate for his age group—appropriate in the sense that it is his main dread. At age forty we all start to worry about losing our memory, and at fifty we are convinced we have. At sixty we begin not to care any more. . .; at seventy we may get sore as hell about it; at eighty we can cause a lot of trouble for everybody because we are so outraged by it. I purposely cited decade birthdays because they are the ages when we review our life situation. As anxiety increases in old age, the symptoms become more and more limited because of the stereotyped and limited expectations of the aged. Thus they have very few symptoms to choose from, and memory loss is the most convenient because it serves so many purposes.[19]

For many old people, memory loss is "a very handy way of tuning oneself out of a totally unbearable situation."[20]

Memory loss, then, is frequently a symptom of withdrawal from present reality and of denial. Dr. Butler speaks of this type of defensive behavior as "selective memory":

The dulling of memory and the propensity to remember distant past events with greater clarity than events of the recent past have generally been attributed to arteriosclerotic and senile brain changes in old age. However, it appears that such memory characteristics can at times have a psychological base, in that the older person may be turning away from or tuning out the painfulness of the present to dwell on a more satisfying past.[21]

Now, this passage was written by the theorist who is primarily responsible for our reevaluation of reminiscence; but it appears so reminiscent of Dr. Lidz that it may well be asked whether Dr. Butler is not himself a proponent of the negative view. Just here, where the issue seems most confused, we are closest to our first substantial clarification.

Dr. Butler would call the kind of reminiscing which is done for the sake of denial "selective memory," whereas Dr. Lidz equates reminiscence solely with selective memory and fails to distinguish between a complex psychological process and one of the aims it may serve. Reminiscence and selective memory, like mourning and melancholia, are terms which distinguish between normative and pathological processes. The negative view never sees in reminiscence anything more or other than a manifestation of denial and impairment. In Butler's view, reminiscence is not reducible to selective memory. Rather, it is the psychological process by which the central life task of old age may be accomplished. Through reminiscence, an old person may review his life, achieve integrity, and face death.

3. MOTIVES OF REMINISCING: DISENGAGEMENT AND NARCISSISM

"Tuning out the present," which Butler and Oberleder speak of as a motivating factor in selective memory, is generally regarded as a manifestation of the "process of disengagement" which Elaine Cumming and William E. Henry observed in their famous and controversial study on aging. "In our theory," they write;

> aging is an inevitable mutual withdrawal or disengagement, resulting in decreased interaction between the aging person and others in the social system he belongs to. The process may be initiated by the individual or by others in the situation.[22]

Whether the aging individual withdraws from society, or, as the "activity theory" asserts, society withdraws from the individual, the outcome is often a decline in social and psychological engagement. "Inner life processes" assume greater importance, and there is a "decreased efficiency in certain cognitive processes."[23]

"Disengagement"—or apathy and rage brought on by social exclusion—may, in part, account for the decline in short-term memory and the "deficit of cognitive ability" which often accompany aging. In discussing the factors which motivate reminiscing, Dr. Arthur McMahon and Dr. Paul Rhudick write that turning away from the present results in a

> disinterest and avoidance of new learning which disproportionately affects memory for recent events. In fact, it has been suggested that reminiscing is an attempt to fill the void created in the present by failing memory. Remote events, on the other hand, were better learned initially, unhampered by the process

of disengagement, and are associated with pleasanter memories of the unimpaired capacities of youth.[24]

Another factor that McMahon and Rhudick discuss is the role which the emotions play in determining what is forgotten and what is remembered.

> The emotional condition of the present: hopes, fears and expectations directed toward the future, determine the appearance in which events of the past are revived or are prevented from reviving (repression). . . . Events which are forgotten presumably under certain circumstances have unexpected revival when a personal situation or phase of life favors it.[25]

Memory, then, not only preserves a sense of self-sameness, but has a creative aspect as well: "it is selective in the direction of. . . creating a sense of personal significance."[26]

Reminiscing may help the aging person maintain his sense of self-esteem by gratifying three persisting narcissistic aspirations, thereby helping him cope with late-life depressions. Bibring, in his theory of depression, identifies the normative narcissistic aspirations as:

> (1) the wish to be worthy, to be loved, to be appreciated, not to be inferior or unworthy; (2) the wish to be strong, superior, great, secure, not to be weak or insecure; (3) the wish to be good, to be loving, not to be aggressive, hateful and destructive.[27]

The capacity to remember events of the distant past with great clarity may be a source of pride and satisfaction, as well as an affirmation of the old person's "biological" achievement: he has survived the accumulating years, with their harsh adversities, to achieve longevity. In this respect, he may view himself, and be viewed by others, as strong and superior, and as possessing extraordinary powers of memory.

It has often been noted that the exercise of the capacity to remember remote events is pleasurable in itself. In explaining this, McMahon and Rhudick cite Freud's comment that when "we do not use our psychic apparatus to fulfill indispensable gratifications, then we let it work so as to derive pleasure out of its own activity."[28]

Reminiscence, like art, may be considered a culturally valuable form of play.

The free play of the mind which reminiscing makes possible may, like the making of art, provide a way of cutting through chronic depression and creating metaphors of self. The many losses which old people commonly endure in late life often bring on a "positive increase in narcissism."[29] The enhanced attention which they pay to themselves and to what is going on within them, their greater self-absorption, which may strike us at times as a disagreeable sort of self-centeredness, may also be responsible for the greater detachment, "contemplativeness," and self-knowledge which we admire.

Now, while increased narcissism in late life may spur some difficult summings-up, some clear-eyed self-encounters, it also "favors the reinvestment of libido in an ideal image of the self in the past."[30] Such ideal images are not to be dismissed as mere fantasies; they may, and usually do, contain and convey a good deal of reality. Like poems, they are acts of the imagination which adhere to, and illuminate, reality. A content analysis of the ideal images that old people create for themselves in their acts of remembering has not yet been undertaken. However, if Bibring's theory of depression were applied to a study of the nondirected reminiscences of old people, the results might confirm what most people who have worked with the healthy aged for any length of time have observed: that their reminiscences are, to a considerable extent, motivated by the wish to gratify the normative narcissistic aspirations. The wish to be loved and appreciated, the wish to be strong and superior, and the wish to be good and loving tend to reappear as recurring themes in many of the stories they tell about their pasts.

4. THE TASK OF OLD AGE

In 1961, Dr. Robert Butler suggested that there is a "universal occurrence in older people of an inner experience or mental process of reviewing one's life."[31] He wrote that

> this process helps account for the increased reminiscence in the aged, that it contributes to the occurrence of certain late-life disorders, particularly depression, and that it participates in the evolution of such characteristics as candor, serenity and wisdom among certain aged.[32]

This formulation was suggested by the results of Butler's NIMH study on normal aging. Forty-seven healthy men, whose mean age was sixty-seven, were studied to determine what medical, personality, and environmental factors contribute to adaptation or maladaptation in the crises of old age. In the six-year follow-up of survivors, Butler reported that "supporting data were found for the hypothesis that, triggered by the approach of death, older people universally undergo a life review leading to various preparations for loss, bodily dissolution, and death."[33]

In everything that Butler has subsequently written or said on the subject, impending death has occupied a central position as *the* motivating factor of reminiscence in the elderly. It is not too much to assert that the profound sense of significance which attaches itself to Butler's concept of the life review derives from his view that it is nothing less than our modern way of facing death, and therefore the spiritual equivalent of older transcendental beliefs and philosophies which taught one "the art of dying." The relation of reminiscing to the act of preparing oneself to face death is insisted upon, for example, in Butler's extemporaneous remarks at a symposium on the "Psychodynamics of Aging," held in 1967:

> I can only reassert that I have repeatedly observed a recurrent process of life review occurring in healthy as well as in troubled old people. . . . My experience has been that all old people have recollections, thoughts of the past, and that they are prompted to question and consider their lives as they have lived them by the realization of the proximity of death.[34]

In 1973, in a cogent review of his own contribution, he wrote:

> In 1961, [I] postulated that reminiscence in the aged was part of a normal life review process brought about by realization of approaching dissolution and death. It is characterized by the progressive return to consciousness of past experiences and particularly the resurgence of unresolved conflicts which can be looked at again and reintegrated. If the reintegration is successful, it can give new significance and meaning to one's life, and prepare one for death, mitigating fear and anxiety.[35]

If, with Butler, we see the life review "as an intervening process between the sense of impending death and personality change and as preparatory to dying,''[36] how are we then to regard motivational factors as disengagement and increased narcissism, whose significance has been stressed by McMahon and Rhudick?

What we are confronted with here are not mutually exclusive positions, but rather differences in emphasis, and we must attempt to find a common frame of reference which will offer a meaningful synthesis of the various emotional and motivational strands we have been pursuing. At the outset, it must be said that Freud's principle of overdetermination allows us to accept a multiplicity of motivating factors, without any irritable reaching after the kind of elegant causal certainty which is possible in the physical sciences. However, psychological theories are not thereby exempt from the requirement of internal self-consistency; and it seems that Erikson's concept of the eighth stage of the life cycle provides the theoretical coherence we are looking for. Erikson's concept, when applied to ''reminiscence theory,'' suggests that it is the need to master the developmental conflict of the final stage of life which provides the primary motivation for reminiscence in old age.

Erikson views the great task of the final stage of life as the integration of all the previous stages of one's life and as the attainment of ''the acceptance of one's one and only life cycle as something that had to be and that, by necessity, permitted of no substitutions.''[39] If the aging person's attempt to give order and meaning to his life experience does not succeed, then ''the lack or loss of this accrued ego assurance is signified by fear of death''—by despair. ''Despair expresses the feeling that the time is short, too short to start another life and to try out alternate roads to integrity.''[38]

Butler's concept of the life review may be regarded as a crucial extension of Erikson's theory; for Butler has postulated the process whereby the old person either accomplishes his task of achieving ego integrity or succumbs to despair. In addition to characterizing the ''mechanism'' of the life review, he has brilliantly extended Erikson's antipodal concept of ''ego integrity vs. despair'' by describing the ''varied outcomes'' of the life-review process in all their ''protean manifestations.''[39] He has devoted as much attention to the ''psychopathological manifestations'' as he has to the ''constructive and adaptive manifestations.''[40]

Like Butler, who has written that the influence of Erikson's concept of the life cycle has been ''deserved and considerable,''[41] McMahon and Rhudick acknowledge Erikson's theoretical generativity. In their view, the adaptational significance of reminiscence can best be understood in the light of Erikson's theory that identity formation is a lifelong development.[42] In saying that reminiscence appears to foster successful adaptation in old age "through maintaining self-esteem [and] reaffirming a sense of identity," they are conceptualizing the significance of reminiscence in Eriksonian terms.[43] And yet, how can the elderly person's "disengagement" and "increased narcissism"—the motivations for reminiscing which they stress—be related to the task of achieving ego integrity? We might begin answering this question by noting that McMahon and Rhudick regard reminiscence as "operating under the control of the ego."[44] They emphasize its conscious, constructive, task-oriented aspect when they say that "affective states in the ego" direct the memory towards "preserving and creating a sense of personal significance."[45]

The increased narcissism which fosters the resurgence of memories that embody a positive or ideal image of the self in the past must also be seen as part of the process of continuing identity formation. If the past is sufficiently charged with experiences that have realistically gratified normative narcissistic aspirations, then it can legitimately provide rich materials for the task which awaits the ego in old age, and the "ideal image" which the ego constructs out of its past may be, in effect, a crystallization of the positive capacities and experiences actually possessed by the old person. However, this will occur only where an increase in the narcissism of a reasonably healthy person plays a part in motivating the life-review process. Butler has provided abundant evidence that the life review of narcissistic personalities—the proud, the arrogant, those who have consciously exercised the power to hurt—must end in despair.[46] And Erikson states that ego integrity is a "post-narcissistic love of the ego—not of the self—as an experience which conveys a sense of world order and spiritual sense."[47]

The process of disengagement may also be related to the ego's task of attaining ego integrity. Erikson, in pointing to a "few constituents of this state of mind," says that ego integrity is

> a comradeship with the ordering ways of distant times and different pursuits, as expressed in the simple products and sayings of such times and pursuits. Although aware of the relativity of all the various life styles which have given meaning to human striving, the possessor of integrity is ready to defend the dignity of his own life style against all physical and eco-

nomic threats. For he knows that an individual life is the accidental coincidence of but one life cycle with but one segment of history; and that for him all human integrity stands or falls with the one style of integrity of which he partakes.[48]

This "portrait" of the possessor of ego integrity summons to mind some of the old people with whom I have worked: emigrants from Eastern Europe in their own and this century's adolescence, they view themselves as the "pioneers" who "planted a new life in America," and their sense of personal conviction about the worthiness of their lifework and the rightness of their traditional life-style gives them a tremendous sense of integrity. It is their sense of identity, their sense of the dignity and value of their own life-style, which in part motivates their disengagement from the contemporary world. It is not to be thought that this disengagement is without pain; but it is undertaken, as Erikson writes, in defense of the dignity of their own life-style. Thus, upholding lifelong practices and beliefs, and customs which they have inherited from previous generations, may often tend to separate them from others in their world, and particularly their own children. However, this is an instance where disengagement is a responsible human choice made for the sake of deeply valued commitments, and cannot be regarded as pathological, although it may, indeed, be sad. The old person may be seen to possess a certain moral passion and a vision of life to which he is unshakably committed; others may find this inconvenient, yet they cannot help but recognize that the passion and the vision are a source of strength.

5. *THE USES OF REMINISCENCE*

McMahon and Rhudick's study of the adaptational significance of reminiscence supplements Butler's concept of the life-review process; and it provides, along with Butler's writings, the theoretical framework and body of knowledge from which later modifications and elaborations have been developed.

Their study evolved out of a multidisciplinary study of 150 veterans of the Spanish-American War which was begun in 1958 at the Outpatient Clinic of the Boston VA Hospital. It was observed that these men, whose average age was eighty-one, were coping unusually well with the problems of aging, and that when initially interviewed they devoted much of the time to reminiscing. "These facts suggested that reminiscing in some way might be related to the success of this group in coping with the problems of later life."[49] Twenty-five of the men were then selected at random, and an hour-long nondirective interview was conducted with each of them. Each sentence of the transcripts was classified according to whether it related to the past, the present, or the future. The men were also rated on the presence of depression and on the degree of intellectual deterioration.

McMahon and Rhudick found that "66 percent of all responses referred to the remote past; 32 percent to the present or immediate past; and 2 percent to the future."[50] There was no correlation between reminiscing and the level of intellectual competence or the decline of intellectual abilities. Further, in the one-year follow-up, they found "that three of the four subjects rated as depressed had died; four of the five subjects rated as suspected of depression had died; and only one of the 16 subjects rated as not depressed had died."[51] In summarizing the results, they write:

> The findings of this study indicate that reminiscing is not directly related to intelligence or to intellectual deterioration and suggest that it is positively related to freedom from depression and to personal survival.[52]

In the first round of interviews, the nondepressed group—and these were the survivors—showed a tendency to reminisce more than the depressed group.

What may well be the most valuable aspect of McMahon's and Rhudick's study is their discussion of the uses of reminiscence. They divided the subjects of their study into four groups "on the basis of their personal use of reminiscence," and they were then able to demonstrate how reminiscing can be useful in coping with the common problems of old age. These problems were identified as "the maintenance of self-esteem in the face of declining physical and intellectual abilities; coping with grief and depression resulting from personal losses; finding means to contribute significantly to a society of which older persons are members; and retaining some sense of identity in an increasingly estranged environment."[53] These problems, together with the fear of death, must be coped with successfully in order for ego integrity to be attained.

It should hardly surprise us that one group enlisted reminiscence in the service of denial: this use of reminiscence has long been recognized. In an article entitled "Ego-Adaptive Mechanisms of Older Persons" published in 1965, denial heads the list of "defenses commonly employed," and the author presents the following case illustration:

> Mr. J., aged 80, is an ambulatory but somewhat feeble patient in a rehabilitation center for the aged, and he displays some mental confusion. Each day Mr. J. tells a staff member stories of his former athletic prowess, comments on his present muscular vigor (even as the nurse is helping him to walk), and requests his discharge from the center.[54]

The relation between remote memories and present denial could not be more vividly demonstrated.

The "case" which McMahon and Rhudick present as typical of the first group also uses reminiscence to deny physical decline:

> I remember the really great players who did everything well. The players nowadays fall asleep on the job. They're good players; but there's something missing there. They. . . don't have the pep the old-time players used to have.[55]

The attitude described here is so nearly universal that it may be said to constitute an archetypal pattern in world literature: both the banishment from Eden and the classical myth of the Golden Age idealize the past and depreciate the present as a time of spiritual and physical decay, of "sin and death." The "golden ager" who projects the symptoms of his own old age—falling asleep, lack of pep—onto contemporary ballplayers was formerly an athlete and clearly identifies with the great players of the past: the days of his own greatest powers become, in fantasy, the great days that are gone. The authors suggest that there is a similarity between this use of reminiscence and the normal adaptive process of fantasy:

> Hartmann has emphasized that fantasy can have positive adaptive elements and contrasts it with dreaming in its attempt to solve the problems of waking life. He maintains that there are avenues of adaptation to reality which at first lead away from the real situation and defines this process as regressive adaptation.[56]

This use of reminiscence, which literally wishes away signs of physical decline, is ultimately a denial of death.

A second group was composed of "several of the subjects. . . [who] seemed preoccupied with the need to justify their lives, and their reminiscences reflected themes of guilt, unrealized goals, and wished-for opportunities to make up for past failures."[57] The use which these "obsessive-compulsive subjects" made of reminiscence was suggested to the authors by Butler's concept, which—as they tellingly summarize it—claims "that the aged person has a need to review his life preparatory to death, and that reminiscences serve to provide the material necessary for this review."[58] But they did not find evidence of life review in the majority of their subjects, who, like the normal elderly population that Busse studied, did not seem preoccupied with a need to justify their lives.

McMahon and Rhudick carefully avoid using the term "life-review process," since Butler's well-defined use of the term denotes a "universal" and "normative" process. It is precisely on these two points that McMahon and Rhudick take issue with Butler:

> It may be significant that the subjects described by Butler (1963) were psychiatric patients who showed evidence of obsessive rumination and clinical depression. Some of the interview material quoted in his article suggests the breakdown of repression and the return of the repressed rather than the organized quality characteristic of the reminiscences of our subjects.[59]

In the article to which they refer, Butler characterizes the life review process as "a progressive return to consciousness of past experiences, and particularly, the resurgence of unresolved conflicts."[60] He would, therefore, have no quarrel with a description of this material as "the return of the repressed." He does, however, add that "simultaneously, and normally, these revived experiences can be surveyed and reintegrated."[61] It is the capacity to reintegrate hitherto repressed material that for Butler, gives this process its normative quality. Further, Butler maintains that the reminiscences may come unbidden, or they may come as a result of a purposeful seeking of memories.[62] This too implies ego control. And Butler himself affirms that "the varied manifestations and outcomes of the life review may include pathological ones."[63] In severe form, these may include anxiety, guilt, despair, and depression; in the most extreme cases, obsessive preoccupation with the past can lead to states of terror and suicide.[64]

The results of the NIMH study on aging which Butler and two colleagues conducted seem to confirm the prevalence of a life review among the normal elderly. Blank, in summarizing the findings, writes:

> At the third point in this eleven-year study, Robert Patterns, Leo Freeman and Butler reported on eighteen of the twenty-three survivors. They state that the survivors often indicated they had reviewed or were still reviewing their lives. Ten of the survivors had been depressed at one of the three times they were examined during the longitudinal studies. Three of these depressions were caused by the despair the subjects experienced while reviewing their lives. The subjects who had reviewed their lives without becoming depressed appeared sometimes to have attitudes that Erikson described as acceptance of one's own life cycle.[65]

This study, while it tends to refute McMahon and Rhudick, in no way may be said to settle the issue of whether the life-review process is or is not normative and universal. This is a fertile issue for further research.

We may, at present, contrast the two views of the life review as follows. McMahon and Rhudick regard a need to review one's life as an indication of a need to justify one's life; unlike Butler, they do not believe that a need for self-justification is the normal fate of humankind, an emotional and spiritual task which awaits all people at the end of their lives. Rather, they regard it as characteristic of "obsessive-compulsive subjects who, we may suspect, have been reviewing their past behavior in the same judgmental and evaluative way all their lives."[66] For them, it is evidence of a lifelong and ongoing pathological process. Butler maintains that "as a natural healing process, it represents one of the underlying human capacities," and that the resolution of intrapsychic conflicts depends upon it.[67] Nor would he view the presence of intrapsychic conflicts as necessarily pathological; insofar as they would be manifestations of an Eriksonian developmental crisis, they would be normative.

Of the group of old men who were clinically depressed, McMahon and Rhudick write:

Depressed subjects showed the greatest difficulty in reminiscing. Their excursions into the past were interrupted repeatedly by anxiety and concern about their physical health, failing memory, personal losses, and sense of inadequacy. They seemed to have given up and to have lost self-esteem.[68]

Bibring has defined depression as a loss of self-esteem brought about by the ego's awareness of its helplessness and incapacity to live up to its narcissistic aspirations;[69] and Butler has found clinical evidence which indicated that the life review process can cause despair in narcissistic personalities. Bibring's "basic mechanism of depression" and Butler's connection of late-life depressions with narcissism strongly suggest one of the factors which may account for McMahon's and Rhudick's finding that the depressed have difficulty in reminiscing. Reminiscence, in narcissistic people, may be inhibited since it would prove too threatening to their self-esteem. Another factor which may cause the inhibition of reminiscence in depression has to do with the way in which depression affects memory. In severe depressions, the memory of well-being is so "decathected," it temporarily disappears, and depressed persons suffer from the delusion of the eternity of their depressed state.[70] Thus, the only memories available are those which exacerbate and enlarge upon the themes of present pain; memory serves as another grand inquisitor which accuses the suffering person the incapacities whose loss he laments. McMahon and Rhudick speculate that the absence of reminiscence in depressed people may be related to the absence of mourning in the "interrupted grief reaction."[71] Further, they find a striking resemblance between mourning and reminiscing:

> The attempt of the ego to cope with loss through repeated recollections, the absorption of the self in this process, the relative lack of interest in the present—these elements are all characteristic of reminiscing behavior.[72]

This is a provocative insight; but the authors' suggestion that reminiscing may be related to "grief work" meets with a seemingly fatal objection:

> The crucial difference is that reminiscence is a process whose function is to deal with attempted *reunion* with past objects,

whereas mourning is a process whose function is to deal with
separation from past objects.[73]

In a brilliant response to this objection, Dr. McMahon points to the
developmental process in which the ego acquires the capacity to
cope with separations and loss through the process of identification.[74] In melancholia, the ego likewise identifies with a lost object
in order to give it up. The capacity to tolerate separation by substi-
tuting a satisfying memory for the missing "love object" begins in
infancy and becomes an important process in identity formation:

> the satisfying qualities of the early object relationship become
> an essential part of the memories of the interaction, providing
> incentive for and giving a satisfying quality to subsequent iden-
> tifications and eventually providing a sense of identity and
> continuity which can exist independently of the object. True
> reminiscing appears to have this quality and function and is
> both a manifestation and reaffirmation of the experience of
> continuity. . .[75]

In old age, mourning often cannot follow its normal adaptive
course. For older persons who have lost their life partners and
lifelong friends, there are frequently no new "love objects" to become invested in. And so McMahon and Rhudick postulate an extended state of mourning in old age; in this situation, reminiscing
becomes "both a manifestation and reaffirmation of the experience
of continuity."

For McMahon and Rhudick, the normative use of reminiscence
par excellence is the one which was traditionally made of it by
village elders, medicine men, oral poets—wise custodians of the
knowledge of the past who were revered in primitive and preindus-
trial societies. They describe their "best-adjusted" group, quite
simply, as storytellers:

> [They] recount past exploits and experiences with obvious
> pleasure in a manner which is both entertaining and informa-
> tive. They seem to have little need to depreciate the present or
> glorify the past, but they do reminisce actively.[76]

The authors cite Hartmann's theory that adaptive behavior, "in the
happiest instances," serves both personal ends and social goals.[77] It

is its twofold adaptive function which gives the use of reminiscences in storytelling its special character:

> The older person's knowledge of a bygone era provides him with an opportunity to enhance his self-esteem by contributing in a meaningful way to his society.[78]

Yet this natural power of old age may be described as a vestigial human function since it can no longer assure old people a place of power and dignity. The various kinds of memory banks in which a technological society stores its knowledge have gone a long way towards making human memory obsolete. However, our culture's reawakened interest in oral histories and in the "roots" which may be found in the reminiscences of older family members may, to some extent, provide a social climate more favorable to old people. While a heightened interest in ethnicity, in "the world of our fathers" and mothers, cannot unmake the structure of modern society, it may to some degree provide the social situation which McMahon and Rhudick so poignantly called for more than a decade ago:

> It seems essential that we find new ways to provide opportunities for [old people] to contribute their knowledge of the past. Anxious relatives sometimes discourage reminiscing behavior within the family group because they consider it a sign of deterioration in their loved ones. It would appear, to the contrary, that this behavior should be encouraged; we should create occasions for older people to reminisce and not expect their reminiscences to conform to the standards of accuracy of historial texts.[79]

Such reminiscences may offer what no historical text can: an enhanced sense of how an individual life is part of a larger historical and cultural process; and hence, they may be the source of a deepened sense of identity and a more profound knowledge of our interconnectedness with the world.

Reminiscence and the Recovery of the Public World

Harry R. Moody

The waking have one world, while in sleep each man turns inward to his own.—Heraclitus

1. REMINISCENCE AND LIFE REVIEW

We know that old people tell stories of the past, but what are we to make of this fact? Opinion is divided here. Aristotle, the hardheaded realist, seems to have no use for reminiscence: he claims that those who retell the stories of the past lack hope in the future. This view is shared by the contemporary philosopher, Simone de Beauvoir, who in her book *The Coming of Age* downgrades any concern for the past on the part of old people: it is an existential misunderstanding, she tells us, not a positive response to old age.

Interestingly, the negative view of reminiscence is shared by many social workers, psychiatrists, psychologists, and counselors who work with the elderly. Their dismissal of reminiscence has much in common with contemporary attitudes that regard the contributions of old people with amused disdain: reminiscence is a tiresome self-indulgence, a preoccupation with forgotten events or people best left forgotten. Above all, it is boring. Reminiscence looks backward and inward. It is best to get on with the business of living.

In a now-celebrated article, Dr. Robert Butler argued that reminiscence is really a form of life review undertaken in old age.[1] Old people, approaching the limits of their life, retrieve memories of the past in order to work through unresolved conflicts—regret, grief,

guilt, unfulfilled dreams. This working through of the memories of
the past is indeed like the work of our dreams during sleep, and it
fulfills a similar psychic function in maintaining our mental
equilibrium in the face of losses, frustrations, and the accumulated
anxieties of a lifetime.

We must be grateful for Dr. Butler's ground-breaking work in re-
deeming the positive value and significance of reminiscence in old
age. His work has taught a generation of gerontologists to see new
meaning, the meaning of life review, in the storytelling of old people. But in reaffirming the value of reminiscence, we must ask precisely what sort of value this is. Return to the aphorism of
Heraclitus: "The waking have one world, while in sleep each man
turns inward to his own." Is the activity of life review a purely
psychological phenomenon, like the dream world of sleep? Or does
it point back in some fashion to the "one world" of the waking?

My argument here can be stated in very simple terms. It is *not* in
our private worlds that we will discover the secret of reminiscence
and life review in old age. Instead, we will find that secret in the
structure of the stories themselves, and in the disciplines of poetry,
history, and autobiography. What is the tale? In the words of *Black
Elk Speaks*, it is the story of all life that is sacred, the story of the
human journey from birth until death. It is a journey through the
public world, the waking world restored by the act of remembrance.

But why does this argument have to be made here at the risk of
preaching to the converted? Let me answer this question by calling
attention to a story, a fairy tale sometimes called *The Hero with a
Thousand Faces*. Those who set off on the human journey seeking
the Pearl of Great Price face many obstacles and dangers on the
way. The Pearl of Great Price is guarded by a dragon, but at the
crucial moment, a Wise Old Man or Wise Old Woman appears to
guide us on the journey. The old person who has traveled on the
journey before can show us, by telling a tale, where the dangers lie.
The telling of the tale is *not* an amusement. It is a guidance—the best
guidance, perhaps the only guidance, that one generation can give
another.

One of the greatest dangers we face is that the whole activity of
storytelling may seem irrelevant. Modern societies discard the past
and thus abolish the possibility of collective memory, the history of
a unified social order in which old people have a function—the function of storytellers, carriers of tribal lore, initiates into the world of
ancestors.

2. THE VANISHING OF THE PUBLIC WORLD

The disappearance of a unified social order in the modern world has been described by a succession of social critics. The threat to the status and role of old age seems clear. One of the most sensitive descriptions of the fate of old age in the contemporary world is given by Christopher Lasch in *The Culture of Narcissism*, in the chapter titled "The Shattered Faith in the Regeneration of Life." Here Lasch touches the heart of the issue. The loss of faith in the continuity of a public world, a world beyond the self, defines our present dilemma. A culture that forgets the past can have no faith in its future. A recent Gallup Poll tells us that, more than ever before, Americans now believe the next five or ten years will be *worse* than the past, that our children will grow up in a world with less opportunity than we have had. Lasch argues that this loss of hope betrays itself in two ways: in the denial of any meaning to old age and in the loss of interest in the future, most tangibly expressed in "uneasiness about reproduction."

> Psychiatrists who tell parents not to live through their offspring; married couples who postpone or reject parenthood, often for good practical reasons; social reformers who urge zero population growth, all testify to a pervasive uneasiness about reproduction—to widespread doubts, indeed, about whether our society should reproduce itself at all.[2]

Our society has become the stage on which we observe the flourishing of the narcissistic personality:

> Because the narcissist has so few inner resources, he looks to others to validate his sense of self. He needs to be admired for his beauty, charm, celebrity, or power—attributes that usually fade with time.[3]

The culture of narcissism then comes to define the fate of old age in a world where remembering the past has lost its meaning:

> [The narcissistic personality is] unable to achieve satisfying sublimations in the form of love and work, [and so] he finds that he has little to sustain him when youth passes him by. He takes no interest in the future and does nothing to provide him-

self with the traditional consolations of old age, the most important of which is the belief that future generations will in some sense carry on his life's work. Love and work unite in a concern for posterity, and specifically in an attempt to equip the younger generation to carry on the tasks of the older. The thought that we live on vicariously in our children (more broadly, in the future generations) reconciles us to our own supersession—the central sorrow of old age, more harrowing even than frailty and loneliness. When the generational link begins to fray, such consolations no longer obtain.[4]

These "generational links" are the life stories in which the older generation unfolds the remembered past; these "consolations" are the love and work whereby each generation participates in a public world surpassing the self: the seeds that will flower and bear fruit in a future extending beyond the limits of our life. This sense of sweetness and sorrow is captured well in John Masefield's poem about the human life course and the succession of generations, a poem titled "The Passing Strange." Its final lines speak of the consolations tied to generational links:

> Only a beauty, only a power,
> Sad in the fruit, bright in the flower,
> Endlessly erring for its hour,
>
> But gathering, as we stray, a sense
> Of life so lovely and intense
> It lingers when we wander hence,
>
> That those who follow feel behind
> Their backs when all before is blind
> Our joy, a rampart to the mind.

The Culture of Narcissism reminds us of a singular and important fact: hope in the future is linked to the task of old age as the guardian of the remembered past. Aristotle, then, was wrong. Reminiscence is *not* opposed to hope. It is the other way around. Reminiscence makes sense only if

> we believe that our memories form a continuous chain from the past into the future, from one generation to the next. Without the idea of generations we would be lost. We would live in a limbo of time made up only of passing scenes.[5]

Accordingly, we are mistaken

> in thinking that [old] people remember only for the sake of the
> past, when in fact old people live and remember for the sake of
> the future.[6]

We will return to this concept of generations, but for the moment
it is enough to recognize this elemental fact about the human condition: our sense of time is collective. Past, present and future,
youth and age, are intertwined, linked in a cycle of generations.
This intertwining of generations is the foundation of the human
world. How could such a primordial fact about our condition be forgotten? This the question that Hannah Arendt addresses in her book
The Human Condition, a work that offers us "dazzling glimpses into
the obvious": an extended meditation on the role of speech, work,
action, political life, and, above all, the meaning of the public
world. This is Arendt's description of that world:

> [This common world] transcends our lifespan into the past and
> future alike; it was there before we came and will outlast our
> brief sojourn in it. It is what we have in common not only with
> those who live with us, but also with those who were here
> before and with those who will come after us. But such a com-
> mon world can survive the coming and going of the gener-
> ations only to the extent that it appears in public. It is the pub-
> licity of the public realm which can absorb and make shine
> through the centuries whatever men may want to save from the
> natural ruin of time.[7]

Time—"the natural ruin of time." Here we have it. "Time held
me green and dying, though I sang in my chains like the sea" (Dylan
Thomas, "Fern Hill"). The singing of the song and the telling of
the tale *must* become public in order to shine through the natural
ruin of time. The common world outlasts any single generation, but
it survives only if it becomes illuminated in a "public realm," and
this act of illumination constitutes the effort of reminiscence and life
review. Reminiscence, by juxtaposing past, present, and future
time, helps us recover this reverence for the public world, and here,
precisely, lies the danger. If the act of reminiscence fails to recover
the public world—fails, that is, to participate in something larger
than a single life story—then reminiscence fails of its larger purpose. In that case, reminiscence becomes merely a "sentimental
journey": an evocation of nostalgia or a flight from the present. By

contrast, the old person who helps the present generation to remember the public world also redeems it from the natural ruin of time, and, for future generations, bestows guidance on the life journey. This, in its highest form, is what reminiscence and life review can mean.

Hannah Arendt's analysis of the public world explains why this understanding of the human situation is in danger of being lost today. The shattered faith in the public world has been replaced by a consumer society, a bureaucratic society, a corporate society—all anonymous worlds in which storytelling and reminiscence have no place. Similarly, the rise of interest-group politics, voter apathy, cynicism about all established institutions—these trends confirm the loss of a sense of sharing a common arena of action. Such passivity and lack of participation in the public world eventually threaten a loss of political freedom.

Politics—or human action in a public world—is at the center of Hannah Arendt's work. In a startling way, she makes clear that political engagement of any kind—from citizenship to revolutionary activity—is connected to being a certain kind of storyteller. Storytelling is an originary, world-creating activity. It is the opposite of living by "fictions": that is, by coagulated social conventions. Storytelling, instead, is a meditation, a reminiscence, an evocation of an individual life journey and a world in which it took place.

Isn't each of us struck silent and attentive when we hear an old man or old woman utter the magic words, "Now I will tell you the story of my life. . ." Storytelling, like political action, is an expression of human freedom, the human capacity to take initiatives, to make a "new beginning." The story is new because each human life, each person born on this earth, is a new beginning. In acknowledging that truth, in recognizing the perpetual capacity of man to "begin again," we glimpse that power in man that constitutes a shared world, a public world which surpasses individuality while disclosing individual freedom as the core of history. "We live life forward but understand it backward," said Kierkegaard. In the act of storytelling, for a moment, these two are one.

3. THE CONCEPT OF THE GENERATION

The concept of the generation is indispensable for the intelligibility of the human life course and of adult life-span development, as psychologists are now beginning to recognize. Sociologists of age stratification have called attention to the importance of the age cohort—namely, the group of all those born in the same year. What constitutes a *generation*, however, is something more than merely formal agreement of birthdate, since a generation is necessarily connected within a circle of current coexistence, as Ortega observes. Being of the same generation, then, means to be of the same age and to have some vital contact.

Take, for example, the generation born in the year 1910. This is the generation that stood at the threshold of adulthood in 1929, the year beginning the Great Depression. Those who were born ten years earlier or ten years later than 1910 would either have been adults or would have been children in the year of the onset of the Depression. In any case, their experience of the history of that time would have been of a different sort. We can see, then, that the "generation of 1910," if we may call it thus, confronted a qualitatively unique series of life tasks, tasks located in a public world whose historical dimensions irresistibly shaped the trajectory of their life. Coming of age in 1929 was a crucial life event that defined the public world of the generation of 1910.

This example leads to our most important observation about Ortega's concept of generations. The same historical event occurs to members of a given generation at the same stage of their life—early adulthood, mid-life, and so on. These decisive historical events lend each generation its distinct biography, its collective historical character, imprinted as that generation moves through historical time. Talleyrand once remarked that those who had not lived before the great Revolution of 1789 could not imagine how sweet life could be. The same has been said of those who came of age before the War of 1914. But all these reflections of generational nostalgia point to a common reality: the discontinuity, indeed, the incommensurability of generations.

Each generation comes of age entering into a shared historical world, a prevailing system of conventions and expectations of normal life. This shared historical culture exceeds any individual life and shapes the contours of its destiny in ways which are unimaginable and invisible until seen in retrospect. We cannot even imagine, said Nietzsche, what future generations will discover in the events that are for us, even now, in the past. Yet a generation can gain some glimpse of these giant historical shapes and can also grasp the scale of the unimaginable that history discloses. As a generation begins to know its own shared historical world, it also begins to recognize its essential unknowability, and this retrospection is the key to the wisdom of a generation. "The owl of Minerva takes flight only as the shades of dusk are falling" (Hegel). It is only in retrospect, in reminiscence, that we grasp our location within an historical succession of generations and at the same time recognize the imprint of that historical destiny within our very personality.

Ortega's concept of generations helps us to see, too, why each generation always misunderstands its successor. When we enter a public world as responsible beings, as adults, it is always a predetermined prevailing historical world. The collective form of life is given to us as a task. Yet we make this task our own, forgetting, eventually, that the world preceded our existence.

Old age is the time when, at last, this life task is seen for what it is. To see a single generation's task is at the same time to apprehend an entire historical world. For the old person who is privileged to see and to communicate this vision of things, it is an understanding of the endurance of the human world, the public world, itself. The self in isolation is ungraspable; so too is the past in its unrepeatable uniqueness. This is why we go over it again and again, why old people tell us the same stories over and over. What Freud described as repetition-compulsion here finds its curative, healing power. "By reliving the passively suffered dream of history, one makes it real and comprehensible, since repeating one's history is a way of mastering it."[8] Mastery through repetition—reminiscence as a kind of dream work, yes, only now we begin to see that this activity amounts to a working through of the past of a whole generation.

Old age reveals a world that preceded our existence and will survive its passing. But *this* generation, this historical consciousness is a precious part of the public world. It is a treasure, the Pearl of Great Price, that must at all costs never be lost. Bearing witness is the final task and the final obligation that must never be failed.

4. REMINISCENCE AND THE IMAGINATION

In the *Phenomenology of Perception*, Merleau-Ponty writes:

> The fountain retains its identity only because of the continuous pressure of water. Eternity is the time that belongs to dreaming, and the dream refers back to waking life, from which it borrows all its structures.[9]

We have come full circle back to Heraclitus at the dawn of Western thought: "The waking have one world, while in sleep each man turns inward to his own." Reminiscence at its outer limit touches dream time, the eternity beyond history, thus arousing in the old person a meditation on the link between waking time and eternity.

The artistic imagination is rooted in the soil of dreams, but its branches reach toward heaven. Like a tree, the imagination bridges heaven and earth. Between the subterranean depths of psychic life and the enveloping transparency of the sky, the air of a common world surrounds all our actions. This bond between dream and public world is also the link between art and history. It was Goethe who understood that these two poles of art and objectivity are never separated and so he gave to his own autobiography the twin title *Dichtung un Wahrheit*—Poetry and Truth.

The moment we separate these two—poetry and truth—we start down a road that leads to the separation between "education" and "therapy." This false separation ends by condemning our deepest wish for meaning to a merely private sense of "life satisfaction," as the gerontologists would phrase it. Once the public and the private worlds are separated, once released from the standards of art and history, the self cannot know itself. Goethe again: "Man knows himself only insofar as he knows his world; he is aware of this world only within himself and he is aware of himself only in this world."

Can I ask, implore, petition, and beg all social workers, therapists, historians, and educators to remember this duality, to remember that "education" and "therapy" are never separated? Do not imagine that this idea concerns only philosophers. Keep the duality in mind in considering each of the methods of practice with older people. Poetry therapy, historical education, drama workshops, group work services all have their uses, but none can grasp the living reality of old age without this act of self-scrutiny called life review. And life review, I have argued, is incomplete without the historical and philosophical perspective provided by the concept of generations.

Each generation reinvents itself, as if for the first time. Too late we discover, each of us, that our invention of ourselves was not new, that it is part of the common tale.

The poet labors in the workshop of the mind, gluing together odd ceramic splinters of the self. The poet works alone, but never by himself. He works without a plan, but guidance is at hand. The product is perplexing, but others will recognize the shape, even when the tools are abandoned and the workshop is in ruins. Reminiscence is the work, but the workshop has no name. If my words have evoked it in you, it was because it was there already.

When reminiscence becomes an act of the imagination, we see the world suddenly populated—and enriched—by the Old Ones, by the Ancestors, those ghostly inhabitants of worlds gone by. I hear their voices outside corridors where old people gather. A *seder* ceremony invokes them, like the Ghost Dance of American Indians, a memorial service, the Tomb of the Unknown Soldier, grandmother's photo album, all ghosts hiding behind yellow clippings in my mind.

I see in the chambers of my memory, I see myself now, a small boy, aged seven, dressed up in Sunday clothes, taken over to Aunt Dorothy's dress shop on the corner of a street in Garden City. How old she was to me then! (In her seventies? Eighties?) Selling dresses to the public, yes, but to me, in memory, incessantly a retailer of dreams. Did I ever have any doubt, then or now, that she was the invoker of Ancestors? All the Seamans, Crafts, Moodys, migrants from old New England. Memories of the Mayflower and the harbor view from Brooklyn Heights—Aunt Dorothy guarded the memories just as she guarded the dream world of costumes, hats, gloves, dresses, all imaginary people, ghosts inhabiting her shop once the doors were locked, and a lonely boy listened to them. Why do I today find myself walking among ruins?

"Your young men shall see visions and your old man shall dream dreams." In my vision I see a new branch of the university growing up in the space between generations. I see the Old Ones gathering and I hear the voices of storytellers as we come together for the work that carries us through our common journey in the public world.

Journey Through the Feminine:
The Life Review Poems
of William Carlos Williams

Bill Zavatsky

I

For some years now the little poem by William Carlos Williams about the red wheelbarrow has been a commonplace in the anthologies:

> so much depends
> upon
>
> a red wheel
> barrow
>
> glazed with rain
> water
>
> beside the white
> chickens[1]

These eight lines have come to be called "The Red Wheelbarrow," a title Williams never gave them, and have further come to serve as an emblem of his poetic art: unsentimental direct observation. If we poke into their history we find that they came into existence as poem XXII (that is the only title) in *Spring and All*, Williams's extended meditation on art and life written in prose and poetry and first published in 1923.[2] What never appears in the anthologies is the gloss Williams appended to the poem:

> The fixed categories into which life is divided must always hold. These things are normal—essential to every activity. But they exist—but not as dead dissections.[3]

When he later adds, "In other times—men counted it a tragedy to be dislocated from sense," it becomes evident that for Williams the definition of "imagination" had much to do with the act of seeing.[4] As relentless an experimenter with language as he was, Williams shows throughout his work an unbreakable faith in the connection between words and things.

"But they exist," Williams asserts of his "categories"—the red wheelbarrow, the rainwater, the white chickens, and the implied beholder of this assemblage—not to mention the beholder's judgment. The visual forcefulness of the poem and Williams's reading of it call to mind C. G. Jung's characterization of the "sensation function," one of the four guides he established for determining how the individual ego relates to its environment.[5] Of these, which include thinking, intuition, feeling, and sensation, Jung defined the latter as "the sum-total of my awareness of external facts given to me through the function of my senses. . . Sensation tells me that something *is*: it does not tell me *what* it is and it does not tell me other things about that something. . ."[6]

Williams's famous homemade banner, "No ideas but in things," qualifies him as the poet of sensation *par excellence* among the classical moderns of twentieth century American literature.[7] "No ideas but in things" is the sensation-function speaking, and indeed Williams's connections with painters (particularly realists like Charles Sheeler and Charles Demuth) and photographers (Sheeler again, and the great Alfred Stieglitz, an important mentor of Williams) are well documented.[8] It is also the judgment of most critics that Williams's strengths as a poet do not lie in the realm of intellectual originality.[9] At his greatest—in the best poems and in the short stories collected in *The Farmers' Daughters*[10]—he is a marvelous recorder (even a documentarist) of urban reality, a writer with an eye for a pretty teenage girl with an acne-scarred face or a yellow flower, bits of green glass mixed with ashes in a hospital yard, or a man-sized piece of wrapping paper tumbling down a street in the wind. His "idea" book, *In the American Grain*,[11] and his thesis-poem, *Paterson*,[12] are jumbled, curious documents, but are enlivened by passages of superb description and convincing dialogue. Nowhere is the contrast between Williams's intellectual pretensions and his native abilities more marked than in his labored essays, where he has his thinking cap jammed on, and the interviews with him conducted by Edith Heal[13] and those collected by Linda Wagner.[14] It is often hard to imagine that the same person produced the essays and the interviews, the distance between Williams's "thinking function" and his rough-and-ready candid responses is so pronounced. We go to Williams, in short, to be *sensitized*: to be given back our abilities to see, hear, smell, taste and touch; to have what the poet Wallace Stevens called Williams's "rubbings of reality."[15]

II

Williams's fine eye and taste for realistic detail ought not to be surprising in one trained for medicine, who spent his entire working life delivering babies and specializing in childhood illnesses. Doctors and sons of doctors—among them Flaubert, Chekhov, Hemingway, and Céline—are no strangers to the literary art. What strikes the reader as unique in Williams, however, is the high degree of development in another function, the "feeling-function," which enables him to imbue what might be leaden reportage with a buoyant, energetic warmth and enthusiasm. "Feeling informs you. . . of the *values* of things," Jung said in the Tavistock Lectures. "Feeling tells you whether a thing is acceptable or agreeable or not. It tells you what a thing is *worth* to you."[16]

Necessarily, a hallmark of the feeling-function is relationship, generally taken to be the province of "the feminine" because of factors which may either be innate or culturally determined. The "jury is out" on this question, a hotly contested one when the issue of "masculine" or "feminine" qualities is debated. However, it is my supposition that family and friendship, the daily give-and-take of human intercourse, child rearing, and the life of the emotions have been dominated by women, at least in William Carlos Williams's lifetime. "Determined women have governed my fate," claimed the poet himself, and his work certainly bears witness to that statement.[17] Some of his greatest poems were written about his paternal grandmother, Emily Dickenson Wellcome, among them "The Last Words of My English Grandmother" and "Dedication for a Plot of Ground." His wife, Florence, affectionately known as Flossie, occupies numerous poems, plays, and the three Stecher Family novels (*White Mule, In the Money,* and *The Build-up*). And his mother, Raquel Hélène Hoheb Williams, appears throughout his work, but nowhere as powerfully as in the remarkable and long out-of-print memoir *Yes, Mrs. Williams*, published in 1959 by McDowell, Obolensky, a company itself "out of print." *Yes, Mrs. Williams* deserves the status of lost masterpiece, in part for the light it sheds on Jung's concept of a "journey through the feminine" toward self-realization, and Butler's concept of a life-review process leading to self-integration.

If Williams's grandmother was a life artist, the survivor he depicted in "Dedication for a Plot of Ground"[18] who fought her way tooth and nail to attain what her grandson called "a final loneliness" in the new world of America (much as he fought the battles of literary and artistic modernism in the "new world" of twentieth century poetry and painting), then his mother, Elena Williams, was the failed artist from whom he inherited his painterly eye and whose still lifes he credited with inspiring his poems.[19]

Williams's mother joined her son and daughter-in-law's household in 1924, when she was seventy-seven. The doctor himself was forty-one. She lived with the Williamses until a few years before her death at the age of one hundred and two—Williams was sixty-six. She and her son had translated Philippe Soupault's novel *Les Dernières Nuits de Paris* (1928) for publication in 1929 and must have accomplished it rapidly.[20] It was not until early in 1936 that they embarked upon the translation of *El Perro y la Calentura*, a short novel attributed to the seventeenth century Spanish author Don Francisco de Quevedo, a copy of which Ezra Pound had left at the Williams house on one of his visits.[21]

It appears that Williams was already in the habit of jotting down his mother's colorful sayings and recollections and that he hit upon the stratagem of translating the Quevedo novel to keep her occupied in her lameness and before cataract operations "would make it impossible for her to see anything for a while. . . . " The note-taking led to the idea of writing a biography of the old woman, using the translation as a framework. In *Yes, Mrs. Williams* he describes the process as:

> A story turning about a story. I shall make it seem as if she told me her life while we were working over the translation, then as if we looked up from that work, speak as if she were telling me about herself.[22]

"Then back to the translation," he added, in a sentence cut from *Yes, Mrs. Williams* but which ends the above quotation as it appears in his "Introduction" to the Quevedo novella.[23]

Williams had selected a story that would be a good catalyst for his mother's storytelling: the book touched on Mrs. Williams's origins. Born in Puerto Rico, her first language was Spanish, a language generally neglected by literary translators until the 1960s.[24] Mrs. Williams seems to have demonstrated "because of her Puerto Rican background" a "bewilderment at life in a small town in New Jersey" and a "detachment from the world of Rutherford," where the Williamses lived.[25] Elena also felt the bitterness of exile and loss when her studies at the Académie des Beaux-Arts in Paris were terminated after three years in the late 1870s upon her father's death, and she was forced to return home. Williams's account of her defeat is deeply moving:

> She was no more than an obscure art student from Puerto Rico, slaving away at her trade which she loved with her whole passionate soul, living it, drinking it down with her every breath—the money gone, her mother as well as her father now dead, she was forced to return with her scanty laurels, a Grand Prix, a few gold medals to disappear into a trunk in my attic, a few charcoal sketches, a full length portrait of herself, unfinished, by that Ludovic [Monsanto, a French cousin], showing her ungainly hands.[26]

"Her heart was broken," wrote her son, perhaps thinking of his own struggles to write and carry on a full-time medical practice, a double life which he was always battling and drawing inspiration from. Finally, the translation gave Williams the opportunity to show the dispirited old woman that her life had not been in vain:

> She is about to pass out of the world; I want to hold her back a moment for her to be seen because—in many ways I think she is so lovely, for herself, that it would be a pity if she were lost without something of her—something impressed with her mind and her spirit—herself—remaining to perpetuate her—for our profit.[27]

But in the final analysis a writer, even one as brilliant as Williams, finds that such a project throws him back on himself; that this kind of experiment in biography is inseparable from autobiography:

> . . . the real story is how all the complexities finally came to

play one tune, today—to me—what I find good in my own life.
She has lived through—and stands as an example of that.[28]

Throughout *Yes, Mrs. Williams* we are given glimpses of the salu-
tary effect that Williams's mother had on his capacity for feeling:

> . . . she has been a good woman. . . good in the sense of be-
> ing a valuable thing to me, when I think about it, a thing of
> value—like a good picture: a sharp differentiation of good
> from evil—something to look at and to know with satisfaction,
> something alive—that has partaken of many things, welcoming
> them indiscriminately if they seemed to have a value—a col-
> or—a sound to add still more to the intelligent, the colorful, the
> whole grasp of feeling and knowledge in the world.[29]

This passage, composed of a series of judgments, constitutes a
marvelous little essay on the nature of feeling function—its activity
of judgment making shading into moral attitude—and how a "dominant" function can flow into less-developed functions. Here, the
transit between sensation and feeling is effected by the powerful influence of Williams's mother: the failed painter, whose "full-length
portrait" we have already seen in the family attic, is valued "like a
good picture."

Elena's memories are colorful, witty, sometimes spicy, irascible,
as well as absorbing from the point of view of language. If the recollections we read in *Yes, Mrs. Williams* were typical of her household
talk, the vividness of her poet-son's use of language can come as no
surprise. Here are a few of Williams's entries:

> Machines? You heard about the little French old lady? They
> were talking about machines and they were saying they were
> going to make a machine to make babies. And she said, No, I
> don't think so, I think the best way is the old natural way!

> In Spain when they would have a religious procession—the
> way they used to be—everyone would take off his hat when the
> Saint was passing. I forget which one it was. But this man was
> walking with his chest out and his hat on. He was a carpenter, I
> suppose—the one that made the figures out of wood.
> Take off your hat, they said to him, see the Saint is passing.
> But he swaggered and paid no attention to them. He merely

said: *Yo lo connosi ciruelo. Ciruelo* is a plum tree. He meant
he knew the figure—or the Saint—when he was still a tree.[31]

You don't know the story? It was one of those big women
who are very pompous and important. She was very com-
manding and mean to her servants. When they wouldn't do
what she wanted them to do quickly enough, she would slap
them. So one day she died and the husband of one of the
women she used to slap all the time hated her so much that,
when he saw her lying there dead, he went up to her and gave
her a hard slap across the face. But she had died suddenly and
when he slapped her he knocked a little bone that was sticking
in her throat and she came alive again. He must have been surprised when he saw that, I can tell you.[32]

I was reading about Pavlova in one of your papers. I didn't
know she was dead so long, about a year. They say she had an
absolutely perfect body, feet and everything—but perfect. I
always feel sorry when someone who is doing so nicely here in
the world has to die.[33]

How it comes back to me! I can see my mother's big bed
here and I had a little crib in the corner, there. At night I would
be frightened and crawl over the sides very, very softly and into my mother's bed, near her. Many times she would wake and
tell me, Go back to your bed. And I had to go back. It was
cruel.[34]

His mother's stories and reflections lead Williams into reveries of
his own:

It is pretty hard for her, but we get along a few pages at a
time. The thing isn't finished yet—we're about at page sixty-
five out of a possible ninety-six and neither one of us has read
it through—but it's interesting in spots. And it gives me a
chance to listen to her especially now when she is extremely
limited in what she can say; I get a chance to take her in, all, a
sort of limited comprehensiveness in what is really an extreme
limitation: her room, the few papers she can decipher, a word
or two of conversation.
The bitterness of old age, lameness, advancing cataract and

the deafness of general sclerosis, of typical expressionless face that even alcohol can no more than flush and half arouse— past even the rancors of regret—old age is intensified by regrets that breed envy, resent solicitudes—

—finally quarrels with that which is nearest, flings what is in the hand aside careless of where it may fall—a sort of too tardy liberation—quarrels with its own infirmities at the last, bitterly.

Even tired of pretense to gain attention—comes out into a sort of clearing, what a man or woman might have been had he or she walked out simply into the street and existed. A horrible caricature of a life that might have been enjoyed, free of pretense, free of care or regret, free of restraint to the unvarnished truth of her condition. It is a discovery—so pathetically limited—

It is the limits that have made it possible, it is the awful finality of it that makes it uniform, universal and beautiful— and dreadfully sad to witness. The return of a sort of pride— real enough. It has a reflection for the brave world—one should know it. Life isn't complete without having witnessed it. It is the end of a life that has a sort of bony flower to the end.[35]

. . . she stands bridging two cultures, three regions of the world, almost without speech—her life spent in that place completely out of her choice almost, to her, as the Brobdignagians to Gulliver. So gross, so foreign, so dreadful, to her obstinate spirit, that has neither submitted nor mastered, leaving her in a *néant* of sounds and sense—Only her son, the bridge between herself and a vacancy as the sky at night, the terrifying emptiness of non-entity.[36]

A childlike innocence, unaffected by age with its maddening mutilations—remains still her virtue. To some it is childish, all the characteristics of a spoiled child—which she was—with her bad temper, fears, vindictiveness of an undisciplined infant. To others an indestructibleness, a permanence in defiance of the offensive discipline which is only a virtue to those who wish to flatten out every rebellious instinct down to a highway levelness for their own crazy facility. Be that as it may she has not given in.[37]

Certainly her life had a definite form and purpose—not by any means sentimental: it was based on somewhat rigid loyalties to the ideal. When she herself was unable to fulfill her desires for personal accomplishment, she transferred her ambitions to her children.[38]

. . .(her) desire to capture the effective male for her uses—high, to be sure! Therefore! Therefore, the excuse for domination seems valid. Men! men that accomplish great things are her ideal. She despised women and especially the modern emancipated woman. She would never understand her brazenness, her pretense of being equal with man and militantly asserting that equality. Look at what men can do! she would say. A woman can't do that.

By which she meant: My men can do that and let any woman try to equal it. But such women are not soft, they drive, they do not comfort—they are too restless, too far gone into the destructive ideal—that is why they are afraid to die: For if their life could have been their end: then they have not lived as they desire.[39]

Can there be any doubt that as Williams speaks of his mother he is also confronting an important part of himself? The interplay of emotion and realization as he ponders her life and impending death suggest another angle to the theory of the life review.[40] Williams's encounter with his mother over the pages of the Quevedo novella shows that it may not be the elderly person who initiates the life-review process at all, that the child or grandchild (or a surrogate figure) coming with questions, at whatever age, has a significant role to play in it. Further, and on the assumption that one's own life and fate are inextricably bound to the lives and fates of one's parents, the life review may be just as crucial and instructive a *rite de passage* for the younger participant as it is for the aging or dying elder. In the course of their work together, Williams became the attending physician at a life review, at once struggling and delighting in the parturition of the image of his mother he would memorialize in *Yes, Mrs. Williams*, in his own mind, and which he would hold up in the book's dedication "To Her Grandchildren." The need Williams feels to preface his mother's remarks with thirty-five pages of what essentially is autobiography suggests that through the stories of our parents and grandparents we shape our own story, our own vision of ourselves. Perhaps one reason for Williams subjecting his mother to the life-review process (without knowing it as such, of course) or Marc Kaminsky arriving with tape recorder to collect his grandmother's tales for *A Table with People*[41] is that the son or grandson must convince himself of his status as an artist by doing homage to the source of his creativity, at the same time as he hopes to convince the mother or grandmother (and himself) that her life and fading stories, her lost opportunities to create, have a continued existence, "one more chance," bearing witness to that "bony flower" of life of which Williams writes. Such an act may be the ultimate affirmation: towards those we love, the insistence that they have not lived without meaning, and our testimony to it.

III

Throughout the Jungian writings on the anima (the psychologist's metaphor for the female component in the male psyche—"the woman within"), stress is laid on the need for men to identify the manifestations of their feminine side and to work toward its integration into their personality. "Vague feelings and moods, prophetic hunches, receptiveness to the irrational, capacity for personal love, feeling for nature, and—last but not least—his relation to the unconscious": these are some qualities of the anima.[42] Shaped by the mother, the character of the anima can either be positive or negative. In the "Introduction" to *Yes, Mrs. Williams*, the poet recorded the negative side of his mother's life experience:

> So grown old—in vain, a woman creates a son and dies in her own mind. That is the end. She is dead, she says. But that vigor for living, clinging desperately to the small threads of a reality which she thought to have left in Paris—the battle is against her. How continue to love in the face of defeat? *Why am I alive? No one can realize what I have desired. I succeeded in nothing, I have kept nothing, I am nothing.*[43]

Here is Marie-Louise von Franz's description of negative anima, which in men expresses itself in "irritable, depressed moods, uncertainty, insecurity, and touchiness":

> Within the soul of such a man the negative mother-anima

figure will endlessly repeat this to them: "I am nothing. Nothing makes any sense. With others it's different, but for me. . . I enjoy nothing."[44]

Those familiar with the interviews done with Williams over the years[45] and with Reed Whittemore's biography, *William Carlos Williams: Poet from Jersey*,[46] know that Williams himself was extremely "moody," subject to fits of depression, and for some years struggled with a serious drinking problem. His first commercially published book, *The Tempers* (1913), carries a symbolic title, "(s)omething that typifies me," he told Edith Heal. "I have always thought of myself as having a temper; I used to lose my temper violently. . . not any more. I was always either excited or depressed." And hard upon this disclosure Williams talks about his mother:

> I was conscious of my mother's influence all through this time of writing, her ordeal as a woman and as a foreigner in this country. I've always held her as a mythical figure, remote from me, detached, looking down on an area in which I happened to live, a fantastic world where she was moving as a more or less pathetic figure. . . . Her interest in art became my interest in art. I was personifying her. . . .[47]

Sour Grapes was the title of a 1921 book of poems. "All the poems are poems of disappointment, sorrow. I felt rejected by the world," Williams said.[48]

Williams's feelings of rejection certainly paralleled those of his mother, cast out of her spiritual home, Paris, and her native island of Puerto Rico. Like the Edgar Allan Poe about whom Williams wrote in *In the American Grain* (1925), Elena was "captured" by her mood, "gave away everything to (her) mood."[49] The difference between mother and son—and it was a crucial one—lay in Williams's acceptance of his "local conditions," which became the cornerstone of his art. Elena's refusal to come to terms with Rutherford achieved symbolic enactment when one winter day in her old age, despite her son's admonitions and neighbors' interventions, she went out upon the icy streets without rubbers, fell, and sustained a broken hip from which she never fully recovered.[50]

The "Prologue" to *Kora in Hell: Improvisations* (1920) stands as Williams's most extensive statement on his "broken style" of composition and a key document in the understanding of the role of the anima in artistic creation.[51] Marie-Louise von Franz writes that the anima functions in a positive way

> when a man takes seriously the feelings, moods, expectations, and fantasies sent by his anima and when he fixes them in some form—for example, in writing, painting, sculpture, musical composition, or dancing. When he works at this patiently and slowly, other more deeply unconscious material wells up from the depths and connects with the earlier material.[52]

Discussing the composition of *Kora* Williams said:

> For a year I used to come home and no matter how late it was before I went to bed I would write *something*. And I kept writing, writing, even if it were only a few words, and at the end of the year there were 365 entries. Even if I had nothing in my mind at all I put something down, and as may be expected, some of the entries were pure nonsense and were rejected when the time for publication came. They were a reflection of the day's happenings more or less, and what I had had to do with them.[53]

Both title and format (the latter drawn from another volume Pound had left at the Williams house) came from Pound. He and Williams

> had talked about Kora, the Greek parallel of Persephone, the legend of Springtime captured and taken to Hades. I thought of myself as Springtime and I felt I was on my way to Hell (but I didn't go very far). This was what the Improvisations were trying to say.[54]

But Williams had been mulling over the theme for some time, and had included a poem called "Sub Terra" in his 1917 collection of poems, *Al Que Quiere!*:

> The idea of the poem is this. I thought of myself as being under the earth, buried in other words, but as any plant is buried, retaining the power to come again. The poem is Spring, the earth giving birth to a new crop of poets, showing that I thought I

would some day take my place among them, telling them that I was coming pretty soon.[55]

"When I spoke of flowers," he adds, "I *was* a flower, with all the prerogatives of flowers, especially the right to come alive in the Spring."[56]

Williams's characterized his method as "automatic writing"; the technique was cultivated by the French Surrealists (although Williams, who hadn't kept up, calls it "Dadaism") to gain quick access to the unconscious mind.[57] Everywhere in his descriptions of his compositional practice, Williams uses phrases like "white heat,"[58] "at tremendous speed,"[59] and he says:

> I didn't go in for long lines because of my nervous nature. I couldn't. The rhythmic pace was the pace of speech, an excited pace because I was excited when I wrote. I was discovering, pressed by some violent mood.[60]

For a poet who confessed that "(s)omehow poetry and the female sex were allied in my mind,"[61] the choice of Kora (identified with seed and corn by the Greeks) provided a crystallization of his feminine side, "buried" as it was in the hard winter months of the physician's profession, waiting for March when it could burst into blossom—"my favorite month," said the doctor.[62] And as Williams begins to discuss the "broken style" of *Kora in Hell*, he immediately proceeds to speak of his mother and her wanderings about the streets of Rome during a sojourn there, this despite the central location of their pension, easy access to trams; he gives any number of reasons why Elena shouldn't have gotten lost, instantly making us aware that he is speaking of his own "wanderings" as he writes, his own jagged patterns of association and sudden mental leaps. Williams continues by showing his mother as she free associates, her conversation moving quickly from one perception to the next, dropping judgments as she goes. Suddenly, however, "there comes a grotesque turn to her talk, a macabre anecdote concerning some dream, a passionate statement about death, which elevates her mood without marring it, sometimes in a most startling way."[63] These associative plunges into the dark waters of the unconscious are the very stuff of artistic creation for Williams, who reflects:

> Thus, seeing the thing itself without forethought or after-

thought but with great intensity of perception, my mother loses her bearings or associates with some disreputable person or translates a dark mood. She is a creature of great imagination. I might say this is her sole remaining quality. She is a despoiled, molted castaway but by this power she still breaks life between her fingers.[64]

This extraordinary passage brings us close to the heart of what Williams seems to have meant by "imagination," a faculty he obviously connected to the feminine in the person of his mother. Half of his first sentence reads like a definition of the sensation function, Williams's strength as a writer. But then the feeling function intervenes, inducing a movement that ranges from vertiginous disorientation ("loses her bearings") to negative value judgments ("translates a dark mood"). Though Elena is a "castaway," her ability to "translate" her moods into action or utterance empower her, giving her domination—the power of judgment making—over life. Williams wrote elsewhere that, for him, "the mood had to be translated into form."[65]

We might then say that, for Williams, the following equation might have held true:

$$\text{imagination} = \text{sensation translated by feeling} \\ \text{into form}$$

or

$$\text{imagination} = \text{sense perceptions translated by} \\ \text{judgment into form}$$

If this formulation has virtue, then Williams's preoccupation with finding the right "measure" for his (and by extension, American) poetry becomes understandable. The act of imagination carries with it a charge of affect, a measurable reaction in the nervous system, and no arbitrary metric system will suffice to register the shocks and calms of his temperament. Each poet must find his own measure, though Williams seemed to feel that his discovery, the "variable foot," could be used by other American poets.[66]

Later in the "Prologue" to *Kora*, Williams asserts that "the thing that stands eternally in the way of really good writing is always one":

the virtual impossibility of lifting to the imagination those things which lie under the direct scrutiny of the senses, close to the nose. It is this difficulty that sets a value upon all works of art and makes them a necessity. The senses witnessing what is immediately before them in detail see a finality which they cling to in despair, not knowing which way to turn. Thus the so-called natural or scientific array becomes fixed, the walking devil of modern life. He who even nicks the solidity of this apparition does a piece of work superior to that of Hercules when he cleaned the Augean stables.[67]

And who had found the means of freeing objects from the stranglehold of "the senses"—why, Williams's mother! And how had she done it? By making judgments about them, by deciding which were valuable, beautiful, ugly, evil, good. And had taught it to her son by her example, which he had now adopted for his method of composition:

> By the brokenness of his composition the poet makes himself master of a certain weapon which he could possess himself of in no other way. The speed of the emotions is sometimes such that thrashing about in a thin exaltation or despair many matters are touched but not held, more often broken by the contact.[68]

The irruptions of the feminine, then, generate a fragmentary, collage style—a style that in Pound's *Cantos*, in Eliot's *Waste Land*, and in Williams's poems marked the first period of literary modernism in our century. The "feminine" impulses locked, like Kora, in the "hell" of the unconscious mind are given free play, and it is no wonder that Williams is the first great poet of the exclamation point in modern American literature. His exclamatory gestures are a sign that he is constantly surprising himself with the material he is able to scribble down as it bubbles from his unconscious. In Williams's work the exclamation point is the emblem of the psychic leap. Jung describes the process as follows:

> . . . only in moments of overwhelming affectivity can fragments of the unconscious come to the surface in the form of thoughts and pictures. . . And, indeed, the things one says when in the grip of an affect sometimes seem very strange and

daring. But they are easily forgotten, or wholly denied. This mechanism of deprecation and denial naturally has to be reckoned with if one wants to adopt an objective attitude.[69]

This *materia*, which others might reject as "silly" or "crazy," is exactly what Williams seizes upon. But because of his firm grip on the "real world" afforded by his senses, he does not falter like Elena nor is he devoured like Poe. Instead he seems to joy in the approach to his intuitive side.

Directly after discussing his mother's "imagination," Williams gives his assessment of modern art. He writes that "the only way man differ[s] from every other creature [is] in his ability to improvise novelty."[70] "Improvise" (the subtitle of *Kora* is "Improvisations") and "novelty" are the important ideas. Improvisation he has already learned how to do from Elena Williams, and certainly her behavior is held up here as the paradigm for modern art—unpredictable, shocking, ugly, naive, eccentric. Her feeling-life is one with what Duchamp and the other moderns are trying to do. And on the heels of this affirmation the poet cries out:

> There is nothing in literature but change and change is mockery. I'll write whatever I damn please, whenever I damn please and as I damn please and it'll be good if the authentic spirit of change is on it.[71]

So does Williams lay claim to the exercise of his imagination, embracing through his mother and the other women important to him his own feminine side, using it as "guide, or mediator, to the world within and to the Self,"[72] the transpersonal factor in human experience which is more than the sum of the personality's components, the goal of what Jung called the process of individuation—the "slow, imperceptible process of psychic growth."[73]

IV

The novels, plays, essays, short stories, and hundreds of poems written by Williams throughout his nearly eighty years testify to an attentiveness to the promptings of the anima extraordinary in American letters, extraordinary not only because of the quantity and quality of his work but also for his devotion to the feminine. There is no other male poet of our century who sings of love as Williams does, who celebrates woman with the passion, tenderness, toughness, and variety he exhibits. This quality did not go unobserved by other poets. Here is a tribute by Harvey Shapiro:

FOR W C W

Now they are trying to make you
The genital thug, leader
Of the new black shirts—
Masculinity over all!
I remember you after the stroke
(Which stroke? I don't remember which stroke.)
Afraid to be left by Flossie
In a hotel lobby, crying out
To her not to leave you
For a minute. Cracked open
And nothing but womanish milk
In the hole. Only a year
Before that we were banging
On the door for a girl to open,
To both of us. Cracked,
Broken. Fear
Slaughtering the brightness
of your face, stroke and
Counterstroke, repeated and
Repeated, for anyone to see.
And now, grandmotherly,
You stare from the cover
Of your selected poems—
The only face you could compose
In the end. As if having
Written of love better than any poet
Of our time, you stepped over
To that side for peace.
What valleys, William, to retrace
In memory, after the masculine mountains,
What long and splendid valleys.[74]

In his last decade, slowed by the strokes which began coming in 1948, Williams nevertheless sustained a large artistic output and accomplished what is perhaps his greatest work, including the three great "life review poems" I would like to touch upon now—"Pictures from Brueghel," from the 1962 volume of that name; "The Desert Music," from the 1954 volume of the same name; and "Asphodel, That Greeny Flower," from his 1955 book, *Journey to Love*.

Every poem can be looked at as a life review—a "criticism of life." All poems, too, deal with what is past, even those in which the author's pen races to capture the living moment. Isn't the act of literary composition—impossible without the act of remembering—justification enough for the practice of reminiscence? What of those old people who don't seem to review their lives, who seem crushed beyond hope, or who circle endlessly among their experiences, unable to see meaning in what they have done? Perhaps the life review is a learned response to one's experience. At least that is what the artist teaches himself to do. And if it is obvious that there can be no element in the life review not present in the life lived, we can say that the artist trains himself from the very beginning to "make sense" out of what has happened to him, trains himself in the art of summing up, in the art of closure. Perhaps the prolonged (and in many cases life long) meditation on the same objects and places is similar to the attentive study of dreams, finally revealing all or more than we could wish to know. The old person whose family complains about the same stories told over and over again isn't very different from the writer who, as critics like to remind us, writes and rewrites the same book over the course of a lifetime. How much choice do we have over what is given us, over those objects and events which become our metaphors of self? But there *is* choice, at least as Williams chose his native Rutherford over medical practice in New York; as he chose life in urban America over the bohemian quarters of Paris or Greenwich Village; as he chose to hone his eye to a sharpness on the local, despite his friend Ezra Pound's jokes in letters from Europe about a culturally backward America.

We can make a quick list of the objects which, over a lifetime of scrutiny, tell us that Williams saw himself in them: the eye; the flower; the bird; the child, especially the girl child; debris, everything from dog-droppings to bits of glass to pieces of paper blowing down the street—the whole spectrum of urban flotsam and jetsam; women of all kinds, from those we have mentioned as dearest to him to daughters-in-law to anonymous working girls glimpsed on the sidewalk in funny poses to whores and arrogant gypsies; the work of art, especially the painting; common American speech, slang included; the poor, the down-at-the-heels, the forgotten and abandoned; the machine, be it fire engine, roaring locomotive, or Ford car; his own persona as "Doc" Williams—and that persona tipping its hat or ready to do battle with his persona as poet; the simple rooms in which he lived and worked. We are what we pay attention to; we are what we remember. Williams's urgent examination of the daily round translates it into the realm of the spiritual.

The title poem of *Pictures from Brueghel*, a ten-part gallery tour through selected works of the Flemish master, gives Williams the opportunity to present a panorama through which to sum up his own career as poet-friend of painters and partisan of modernism in painting.[75] Brueghel's modernity, Williams suggests, was like his own: the genius for rendering his own time and place. We have none of the more surrealistic works of Brueghel represented here, and the emphasis (whether in the foreground or background of Williams's description of each painting) is always on the act of seeing. The artist's eyes, says Williams, talking of Brueghel's self-portrait (a genre in which the doctor also specialized) are "red-rimmed/from overuse he must have/driven them hard,"[76] enjoying his joke, this writer who spent hours working in the fixed-up study of his attic, who "used to come home and no matter how late it was before I went to bed I would write *something*,"[77] and who was also famous for yanking his typewriter out of his desk and banging away between patients, or pulling his car to the side of the road to scribble on a prescription pad—"no time for anything but his painting," Williams again jokes.[78] In "Pictures from Brueghel," Williams paid homage to all he had learned from the visual artists, classic and modern, who literally taught him how to see his own world with his own eyes. It stands as his great summary poem on the gift of sight, the sensation function at the heart of Williams's poetic intelligence.

"The Desert Music," the crowning poem in what I believe is one of the finest books of American poetry ever written, a masterpiece of concision and design, operates in more complex ways than the Brueghel poems.[79] On the surface it consists of the fragmentary narrative of a walk into Mexico across the international boundary at El Paso, the events of an evening spent in Juarez, and the return across the bridge, upon which, coming and going, Williams stumbles across "a form/propped motionless,"[80] nothing less than the shadow of death. Good doctor and poet, only he stops to inspect it, as if he anticipated his own end. Except for that specter, "The

Desert Music'' recapitulates the sensation function and its glories: art made out of what is given one through the eye, the ear, the nose, the mouth, the hand. The poem stands, too, as a summary of all he had taken—and himself made in poetry—from the avant-garde artists: fragmentation, collage juxtaposition, abandonment of transition, sudden shifts between imagery and abstraction. It is almost what came later to be called a "found poem," and in its touching upon the "high spots" resembles a travelogue. The witty point Williams makes about his own "broken style" and modern art projects his theory of composition onto an archetypal backdrop:

> I am that he whose brains
> are scattered
> aimlessly[81]

Some thirty years after *Kora* Williams justifies his "leaps" by invoking another myth, that of Orpheus, the first poet, maybe the first collage (or collaged) artist, torn to pieces by maddened women.

The poem ends in a great avowal that bursts from his lips when he realizes that the music of the Mexican streets and cheap strip clubs is the same "protecting music" of his verse, the same music Orpheus made:

> I *am* a poet! I
> am. I am. I am a poet, I reaffirmed, ashamed
>
> And I could not help thinking
> of the wonders of the brain that
> hears that music and of our
> skill sometimes to record it.[82]

Again Williams celebrates the role of the senses in his art, but because of his encounter with the shadow on the bridge, he knows he sings beneath a cloud. The shadow of death has fallen across his faculties, the series of strokes which impaired his speech, severely curtailed his activities for periods, and even made it necessary for him to learn to read again. One might guess that Williams thought *The Desert Music* would be his last book of poems. "The descent beckons/as the ascent beckoned," its first poem begins and opens outward into what is probably Williams's most penetrating statement about reminiscence:

                    Memory is a kind
of accomplishment,
            a sort of renewal
                    even
an initiation, since the spaces it opens are new places
            inhabited by hordes
                    heretofore unrealized,
of new kinds—
            since their movements
                    are toward new objectives
(even though formerly they were abandoned).

No defeat is made up entirely of defeat—since
the world it opens is always a place
            formerly
                    unsuspected. A
world lost,
            a world unsuspected,
                    beckons to new places
and no whiteness (lost) is so white as the memory
of whiteness.[83]

The other poem in *The Desert Music* which must be mentioned,
however briefly, is the extraordinary "For Eleanor and Bill Mona-
han."[84] Presumably dedicated to Irish Catholic friends of Williams,
who was not himself a Roman Catholic, it begins with the exclamations: "Mother of God! Our lady!/the heart/is an unruly Master."[85]
Here is Williams's poem to the Great Mother, the vessel of the eternal feminine, the anima power to which men ought to submit themselves and be "the flowers/spread at your feet."[86] He writes:

I do not come to you
            save that I confess
                    to being
                    half man and half
woman.[87]

and ends:

The female principle of the world
            is my appeal

> in the extremity
> to which I have come.
>   *O clemens! O pia! o dolcis!*
>   *Maria!*[88]

That Williams sees himself in the figure of Tiresias, the blind seer
of Greek mythology, who as an old man was changed into a woman
when he disobeyed the gods, is an important revelation. For in the
process of individuation, as one moves beyond anima involvement,
"the unconscious again changes its dominant character and appears
in a new symbolic form, representing the Self, the innermost
nucleus of the psyche."[89] Tiresias is just such a figure, transcending
mere male and female knowledge and pointing to a wholeness that
reconciles psychological opposites. There is also an implication in
the poem that even the heart, in Hindu thought the seat of the ego,
must be abandoned in the search for transcendence.

The third of what I am calling Williams's "life review poems" is
"Asphodel, That Greeny Flower," with the exception of his epic
Paterson the poet's longest poem.[90] Cast in three "Books" with a
"Coda" and running to nearly thirty pages, it is a love song spoken
by the poet to his wife and a meditation on the power of love, again
in the shadow of death, a death which faces not only Williams but all
of civilization—nuclear extinction. It is not death itself, however,
even by the atomic bomb, that Williams fears; rather it is acts which
kill the spirit:

> If a man die
>   it is because death
>   has first
> possessed his imagination.
>   But if he refuse death—
>   no greater evil
> can befall him
>   unless it be the death of love
>   meet him
> in full career.
>   Then indeed
>   for him
> the light has gone out.
> But love and the imagination
>   are of a piece[91]

Williams suggests throughout the poem that he is writing from somewhere beyond life. "We lived long together," he tells Flossie,[92] and

> I cannot say
> > that I have gone to hell
> > > for your love
> but often
> > found myself there
> > > in your pursuit.
> I do not like it
> > and wanted to be
> > > in heaven.[93]

The tone is that of the *vates*, both urgent and detached. Among Williams's work it has almost a biblical ring, a "wisdom poem" full of sweeping statements about life and love, a mode more thoughtful, more abstract, but exhibiting just as much attention to close detail as his other work. "Asphodel" is an altogether breathtaking performance. Again the poet invokes the image of Kora, locked in hell, and Orpheus, who journeyed there to find his Eurydice—both metaphors of the artist's relationship to his anima and related to the title of the last great book published in Williams's lifetime, which houses "Asphodel"—*Journey to Love*. The path to love is arduous, a journey; the book epitomizes what the poet has learned as he has traveled toward love; a kind of purification must take place along the hard road of life before one can fully love. Part of the tone of the book arises from its attitude of curiosity about death, that of the physician who once carried the corpse of a baby across New York City in a suitcase, who, like Tiresias, has seen both sides:[94]

> Approaching death,
> > as we think, the death of love,
> > > no distinction
> any more suffices to differentiate
> > the particulars
> > > of place and condition
> with which we have been long
> > familiar.
> > > All appears

as if seen
          wavering through water.
                    We start awake with a cry
of recognition
          but soon the outlines
                    become again vague.[95]

This passage recalls the final stanza of "The Last Words of My English Grandmother," with the "particulars/of place and condition" subtracted:

          What are all those
          fuzzy-looking things out there?
          Trees? Well, I'm tired
          of them and rolled her head away.[96]

Williams alludes to other poems of his in "Asphodel," including more recent ones, illustrating that the women of his family had even prepared him for the manner of his death. And a good deal of the beauty and emotional resonance of the poem stems from the farewell Williams seems to be making to sight, smell, and touch, as he utilizes them with perhaps greater clarity than he had ever done before:

When I was a boy
          I kept a book
                    to which, from time
to time, I added pressed flowers
                    until, after a time,
I had a good collection.
          The asphodel,
                    forebodingly,
among them.
          I bring you,
                    reawakened,
a memory of those flowers.
          They were sweet
                    when I pressed them
and retained
          something of their sweetness
                    a long time.[97]

The image of the asphodel,[98] and flowers in general, dominate this wonderful poem, which Williams fittingly calls a "last flower" and offers to his "flowerlike" wife.[99] From the beginning of his work, Williams's attention to flora (and we ought here to remember that "Florence" is a flower-like *name*) symbolizes the attention Williams lavished on art and life, as physician and poet. He drew the art of poetry closer to everyday life in his work. In his hands the poem, like the flowers, becomes an art event accessible to all, not a hothouse product. The flower in this poem is also a life-death symbol, a continual object lesson in growth, change, frailty, decay, persistence, the need for love and nurturing. In the image of the asphodel, Williams binds his entire life as a creator, fusing in a metaphor the wisdom to which his journey to love had brought him.

Old People, Poetry, and Groups

George Getzel

At first glance, poetry groups and old people are an unlikely combination with poor prospects. Popular wisdom informs us that you can't teach an old dog new tricks. For that matter, even if an elderly person has the capacity to compose a poem, of what value is this activity?

A writer, by asking an old person to make poetry, issues a challenge to share personal thoughts and assure his survival beyond the grave. Each poem is a touchstone of remembrance, something that will remain behind. Writing a poem is inextricably tied to an encounter with the boundaries of time that surround every human life.

Rollo May suggests humanness is defined by the creative life: "the essence of being human is that, in the brief moment we exist on this spinning planet, we can love some people and some things, in spite of the fact that time and death will ultimately claim us all, that we yearn to stretch the brief moment to postpone our death."[1] Old people in writing groups learn about each other's individual efforts to leave behind tracings of their past, visions of the world they created and the world that remains for others to create. Through their poems, they share their legacy with the writer and their children and grandchildren or unknown persons of generations to come. The writing affords them an opportunity to discover or rediscover in themselves the larger life of their generation and their own quest for generativity.

The writer and the old people face many obstacles as they develop ways of writing poems together. Obstacles occur in the intertwined creative processes of writing poetry and becoming a group. Both poetry and groups are work and each reflect individuals' drives, wishes, and values. The poem and the group are tangible objects or "thought-things,"[2] and each represents an effort of individuals to grant permanence to valued ideas. When poetry and group interaction occur together, enhanced stimulation and reinforcement of purpose are possible.

193

Four obstacles must be overcome by the writer and the group. The first obstacle the old people and the writer face is a persistent, largely unavowed doubt that the aged can write poems. Their distrust of themselves may be so intense and pervasive that these feelings are inaudible to them, and denied. Many old people doubt themselves as workers and distrust those who view them as capable. Kenneth Koch, in speaking of his workshops with the impaired elderly in nursing homes, suggests that the writer can demonstrate his belief in group members' capacity by "always paying attention to the text, and especially the aesthetic qualities of the text, rather than to the person who wrote it."[3] This approach would obtain whether the group was discussing the work of Keats or a group member's poem. Koch implores others not to use "a kind of falsely therapeutic and always reassuring attitude."[4] The writer should be aware of the hidden hurts of making nice and making do. Sadly, many activities with the aged are governed by the myth of aging as a "second childhood." If we subscribe to a childlike image of later adulthood, we see the group members' depression and helplessness as confirming a pervasive societal distortion of old age. The writer must be particularly aware of the tendency to infantilize the elderly when he is angry with the group because they do not perform according to his standards of production.

The writer expresses his appreciation of members' efforts, and he assists their understanding of poetry by slowly and gently opening up hidden powers of language in their own poetry. The group members in turn deepen their appreciation, and they influence each other's work.

Appreciation comes in many forms—quiet recognition, dismay, anger, applause, silence. The job of the writer in the group is to acknowledge appreciation in whatever form it comes. Slowly the writer responds through his understanding of the text and of the feeling and thoughts shared by group members. Ultimately the writer and the old people are able to show they care about each other through their work together. Caring is appreciation and contribution intertwined.

The second obstacle is the writer's confrontation with the group members' hopelessness. He hears old people ask, "Why do you want to work with us?" Why would you expect us to do something valuable?" Sometimes they ask, "How can you listen to old people's problems all the time?" These questions are frequently asked impulsively, with painful uneasiness. At these moments, denial or flight can be quite appealing options.

We hear these questions as a confrontation. We must respond or lose the contest. Why do we feel challenged? To the extent that we have identified with their hopelessness, the questions sting and hurt. At these powerful moments of inquiry, old people are asking an unavowed question, not in the style of confrontation, but plaintively: "Despite the way I look to myself and you, do you see me as a whole, enduring human being, still facing life's challenges?" We succeed when we are prepared to acknowledge the question and say yes.

The third obstacle is related to the reluctance of the writer to acknowledge the sources of pain and tragedy in poetry and in group discussion. The reluctance in its simplest manifestation occurs in the first moment of contact between the writer and the group. The writer may see only withered limbs, creased faces, and the ragged outlines of stooped bodies. When the writer says "Let's write poetry. I'll help you," he is agnostic and visionary in the same breath.

The discomfort felt by the writer is generated by old people's oft-told tales of pain, illness, and death. Upon closer examination, the writer can sometimes hear rage at him for being young and whole. Frequently seeing the denegerative conditions in the elderly induces fear and guilt. The writer may seize the initiative and not allow in or hear their pain. When this occurs, both group members and poetry suffer. Sometimes the group members will be good enough to say to the writer that he is not listening. Often group members believe that they cannot risk the writer's reaction.

Pain, illness, and death, the frequent companions of the aged, must be accepted as subjects for poems and group discussion. At the same time this content cannot be forced in order to have "depth." Contact with human finitude cannot be orchestrated; it is a face-to-face reality for group members. Moments will come when the winding sheet becomes unraveled, and ultimate prospects are considered by group members. Paradoxically, by understanding the necessity of discussing the inescapable problems of human existence and the imminence of death, the writer helps members become enlivened. Through discussion of these concerns in the group, members can become more acutely aware of the moment of their own existence and that of others.

Writing poems in groups makes members think of themselves in terms of other old people. Together group members explicitly address the submerged questions of old age: What shall I do in the time remaining? What does it mean to live, and to live this long? These themes are also found in their poems. The use of reminiscence in poetry is evidence of the use which old people make of the past. They speak of it to address the question of the meaning of life's drawing to a close. Often reminiscence is accompanied by apocalyptic or idyllic visions of life's ultimate purpose.

Embedded in both individual and collaborative poems are powerful wishes and fears, and efforts to understand and master worlds past and worlds to come. Sadly, questions of ultimate meaning may not have a place in the everyday lives of the old. The group, with the assistance of the writer, legitimates the right of each member to express the unspeakable. Forlorn and despairing spontaneous utterances are taken down by the poet, and returned to the group as a poem, or they may be evoked by way of a response to a poem. Insight and catharsis are confirmed in silence or in communion. Kaminsky says that the writer "is not afraid of identifying feelings which politeness bans, and identifying with persons whom society habitually shuns. He has found ways of making large acceptances which run counter to the received opinions of the day; and where social convention does not fit what he feels and perceives, he has the temerity—it is born of necessity—to oppose his culture along the scrimmage of his choosing."[5] Koch writes in a similar vein: "In poetry one can talk about feelings without thinking about the listener's reaction, without worrying too much about looking good, without making anyone else feel bad (guilty, overly concerned) and without the expectation of someone's feeling an obligation to cheer one up. One's feelings, which are strong things, can, even when they are unhappy feelings, go into making something beautiful, which no one would be distressed to hear."[6]

The fourth obstacle faced by the writer is brought about by his giftedness, his knowledge, and his intuition. He may feel a special urgency to demonstrate expertise at moments of frustration, anxiety, or exhilaration; but he would do so at the expense of group members. The writer may not readily see this as overprotectiveness and as preempting the participation of group members. It may appear to him that the group members are benefiting from his gift of knowledge or insight, but they and their poetry suffer because he in fact has stopped listening. The writer may encourage mimicry and banal writing. And because he has ceased to be deeply attentive to the changing interactions and reactions of group members, magic moments are lost.

The group itself is a special universe comprised of elderly people who reveal varied aspects of themselves through their writing and their actions. The only constant thing in a group is surprise and uncertainty. The task of the writer is to provide group members with ways of apprehending uncertainty in the group and in their poetry, and ways of turning surprises into a source of energy and closeness. The writer uses collaborative and individual writing "assignments," as well as readings and objects of beauty, to encourage the old people to risk their lines of poetry in the group. The writer must allow group members to bend these structures to fit changing ideas, feelings, and needs. Occasionally the writer identifies the "unspoken" wishes of members and relates them to the poetry and the group task. A dream or premonition, for example, is a rich storehouse of symbols that may transcend its private meanings. As the writer acknowledges and explores uncertainties, group members develop the confidence to investigate a wide range of issues and artistic forms.

In time the group will develop traditions and forms of dealing with the writer. The aim of the writer ought to be to encourage group members to decide how they want to use his expertise. The writer must openly recognize the group's unique ways of handling its problems. Once this is done, the writer can allow members to express their disagreements and trust the group's particular style of dealing with conflicts.

Kaminsky sees poetry groups establishing a sense of fellowship: "One of the most vital things that happens in the poetry group is that several individuals discover that they are not alone in feeling as they do about their parents or their children, or their husbands; that they are not alone in their fear, or their anger, or their envy; that they are not alone in their self-involvement, or their sense of loss, or their generous acts; that they are not alone. Barriers come down, and the sense of isolation gives way to a sense of community."[7]

The world, as we know it, is impersonal and cruel. People feel mutilated by being put into categories and turned into statistical trends and probabilities. We are given few opportunities to wonder about our place in the world or to be in awe of the complexity and the uniqueness of a single human life. Through poetry, an old person can sift through life's mysteries, seek perspectives, and sanctify his unique existence.

Poetry encourages reverie and gives permanent form to fleeting thoughts and feelings. Reverie is sparked in the reader. Poems are signs of indebtedness, statements of existence, to be heard and remembered. At their best, poems touch us in such a way that they are not only heard and understood but transfigure the reader, and we are grateful. The recognition poetry offers heightens the sensation of life.

Abraham Heschel, the religious philosopher, writes: "Beyond all agony and anxiety lies the most important ingredient of self-reflection: the preciousness of my own existence. To my own heart my existence is unique, unprecedented, exceedingly precious, and I resist the thought of gambling away its meaning. . . . In actual lives of actual men, life even when felt to be a burden is cherished deeply, valued supremely, accepted in its reality."[8]

Within the group, old people frequently try to create beauty as a means to combat the wounds made by the inevitable losses of the passing years. Flights into beauty—mountains, flowers, blue lakes, cherubic grandchildren—are a balm that enables them to sustain the loss of vigor, spouse, children, friends, home. Poems and group discussion also abound in themes of sadness, desolation, sudden death, lingering illness, trembling.

Upon close examination of old people's writing, we see powerful alternations of despair and melodic bursts of hope; their poems fathom areas of dirt and dread and come back to the pulse of life. An old woman in a group speaks of

Crazy Wisdom

I find good things
in situations where others complain
No one thing is ugly
Even a dirty thing
has beauty in it.

If I see a colony of ants
people would say Yuch, those worms!
But I stand there and watch them
and watch them
You'd be surprised
what they do—so much work, so lovely!
Is there something wrong with me?

I don't think it's real
I don't see the dirt
There's something bigger than that
I see the bigger thing.—Lilly Palace[9]

Another woman dreams of old places:

Sioux City, Iowa

No matter where I go or what I do, my mind goes
back to Sioux City, Iowa.

My friend gave me a flower from her yard.
Immediately I traveled back to Sioux City, Iowa,
but to one certain spot. The field—it will
always be the dandelion field.

There were row upon row of wild grasses rippled
by the summer breeze. Wild flowers grew in abundance.
The smell of wild clover was all about me. Tall
sunflowers looked at me with dark beautiful eyes.

My friends and I sat hidden by the tall grass.
We made jewelry for ourselves out of the dandelion
stems. We braided bracelets and necklaces for
ourselves.

No matter what happens in my life, I go back
to the dandelion field. It is a place of hiding
from the harshness of the city in which I live.—Leah Cahn[10]

The central approach of the writer must be to help old people turn
the problems of old age into tasks for the group and themes for its
poetry. The world for group members becomes at once a problem
and a task. Group members expose their private problems, and each
member is challenged to search for solutions to struggles he cannot
escape.

Writers and professionals in the aging field have an opportunity to
deepen their understanding about human aging through poetry
groups. Deeply meaningful experiences await all those who are
prepared to accept the challenge. Our lives can be enriched by the
words old people leave behind through writing. Their wish for im-
mortality is addressed, and their legacy is protected by our efforts.
We may also begin to see this work as preparatory to our own
frightful and clumsy mastery of the aging process. Old people are an
emblem of our destiny.

Realities of Aging:
Starting Points for Imaginative
Work with the Elderly

Susan Miller London

Recently, programs to fulfill older people's expressive needs have sprung up in the form of creative arts workshops. A personal and painful experience made me interested in training the artists who teach these workshops. First, the experience.

In 1976, the Theatre for Older People was formed as a project of the Joseph Jefferson Theater Company, a professional off-off Broadway theater housed at the Little Church Around the Corner. Because I was eager to start the project, I decided not to work with older nonprofessionals who would need training. Since the Joseph Jefferson Theater wished to provide a community service, they made available their professional actors and staff, as well as their facilities.

The idea behind my forming this theater was to present original plays on issues of aging to audiences of older people. After each performance, there was a group discussion: the play served as a springboard for the older people in the audience to express their own thoughts and feelings. These discussions were led by professionals in the fields of gerontology, psychology, social work, and education. I saw the project as having recreational, educational, and therapeutic goals.

For the opening production, we put together a revue based on the writings of older people in the psychology classes and human relations workshops I had been teaching. The writings dealt with the memories, experiences, and concerns of those who were growing old. We called the revue *Prime Time: A Celebration of Aging* because we focused mainly on material that portrayed positive aspects of aging.

In addition to our five older actors, two men and three women whose ages ranged from about sixty to eighty, we engaged a young woman to direct the play. She had come highly recommended, was experienced, and seemed sensitive to the material and to the goals of the project.

The first few rehearsals made us optimistic. The director had a good rapport with the actors, and she seemed to have an interesting theatrical concept for the text, which was a loosely structured series of writings. Breathing a sigh of relief, I went about doing all the other things necessary to get a new production and a new project off to a good start. I did not attend rehearsals, but from time to time talked to the actors who were very pleased with their progress and with the work of the director. A week before the opening, I attended a rehearsal and was stunned by what I saw. *Prime Time* was no longer a theater piece, but resembled a radio show in which a group of old people sat on wooden boxes and stood up when they had a line to say. From time to time, the men moved around the stage a bit, but these movements were rare. As I watched the rehearsal, I thought it looked like a group of people sitting *shiva*. (In the Jewish mourning ritual, those who are grieving sit on small hard boxes or benches.)

I tried not to let the actors see my dismay, as they were obviously enthusiastic about their work. When I spoke to the director after the rehearsal, I told her that the play was static, without theatrical life, that it reminded me of a radio show. She did not seem too surprised by my comments. She told me that given the ages of the actors one could not expect much more. To illustrate her point, she said that one of the actors—a woman in her seventies—could barely walk across the stage without hobbling. I suggested that this particular actor would have no problem if she took off her three-inch high-heel shoes. Unconvinced, the director went on to enumerate the actors' difficulties, and she would not move from her position: no extensive changes could be made; the actors would be unable to learn new lines, cues, and stage directions because of their age and our time limits.

Five days before opening, there was no imminent solution, and the pressure was mounting. I seriously considered canceling the show. However, in the usual illogical way of most theater projects, the situation resolved itself. The executive director of the Joseph Jefferson had a dream about her deceased father; she felt the dream told her that if the show went on in its present state it would irreparably harm the project. When the director still refused to make any changes, it was mutually agreed that another director would have to take over.

The actors were furious! When we announced the change of director, two of the actors quit on the spot. One of them threatened to report us to the Episcopal Diocese for immoral conduct. After their dramatic exits, there was a moment of silence; then an eighty-year-old actor spoke for the remaining cast. She said, "I'm outraged by what you've done. We were all pleased with the director and with our work. How can you expect us to do a show with a new director with only five days to opening?" She paused—the tension was unbearable. "But since I've worked with you before and always found you to be more than fair to actors, I will give you and the new director a chance. If I feel the new direction of the show is better, I'll stay. If not, I too will quit after tonight's rehearsal." The other two actors agreed with her position. Holding our breaths, we started the rehearsal with the new director.

Since the new director had been called in a few hours before the rehearsal, he had little time to prepare and had to improvise during the rehearsal, making the situation even more tense. At the end of the rehearsal, we were pleased and excited with the changes. The radio show was transformed into a revue which had music, movement, and simple dance routines. The actors conferred, and the eighty-year-old spokesperson said that although they were probably crazy, they all agreed to stay. The show would go on! But we soon discovered it would have to go on with only four characters and with one character played by a man in his forties, since we could not find professional older actors on such short notice.

The changes meant five days of continuous, hard work: the unlearning and relearning of lines, cues, stage business, and the learning of the added movement and dance. By opening night—a benefit performance to raise money for the project—the actors had mastered the new material. The audience was carried away by the life, energy, and professionalism of the older actors. When the curtain came down, they cheered. Perhaps even more than the play itself, the older actors projected the message to the audience—largely composed of younger people—that aging was not synonymous with illness and decay, but could be a time of growth.

Often I have thought of this experience and regretted that I had not thought to discuss the aging process with the first director. So much difficulty and unhappiness would have been avoided.

My interest in training people who work with the elderly in the arts dates from this time. Subsequently I have taught the training seminar of the New School's Creative Arts Center for Older Adults.

In the training seminar I have had the opportunity to explore some of the issues of concern to those who teach arts workshops to older adults.[1] Following are some of the points I have found to be of importance.

1. ATTITUDES

A 1975 Harris Poll for the National Council on the Aging, replicating twenty years of studies about attitudes toward aging and the elderly, found that both young and old in our society view most people over sixty-five as not very bright or alert, not very good at getting things done, not very physically or sexually active. In our youth-oriented and age-segregated society, it is not unlikely that many artists and teachers have negative attitudes toward the elderly. In a workshop situation, the teacher's attitudes and expectations have a direct bearing on the student's creativity, both on the process and the outcome. Thus, an examination of attitudes toward aging and older people seems to me to be the starting point for anyone working in the creative arts with the elderly.

Unrealistic attitudes—whether positive or negative—can be problematical to the teacher. In my early teaching experiences with older adults, I had a "rose-colored" view of the elderly which got me into trouble. Initially I accepted a job teaching older adults solely because I needed the work. Having had a stormy relationship with a difficult and hypochondriachal grandmother, I had little love for the elderly. In fact, I viewed all old people as cranky, depressed, and depressing. My first group of older people in Bedford-Stuyvesant was a delight, and I experienced a total reversal of feelings. With a new convert's zeal, I thought older people could do no wrong. Given my low expectations of their abilities, whatever they did seemed wonderful to me. Feeling that my mission was to help the elderly, I found myself involved in inappropriate relationships and situations in which I was often exploited. It took a hostile ninety-three-year-old man in a human relations workshop to shock me into reality. Rude and abusive, Mr. G. really knew what "put-downs" would get to me. Finally I ran out of excuses for the negative behavior he constantly directed at me. I realized that it was not possible to like all older people: they were individuals with good and bad characteristics. Extending this thinking, I began to see that their accomplishments and talents varied, and I was wrong to deem anything they did as wonderful because they were old. When I began to see older people realistically, it became clear that they did not have to be the recipients of my "bounty." After a period of adjustment to this new way of thinking, I began to enjoy my work more and felt more effective as a teacher.

Identifying and understanding one's attitudes toward the elderly are important first steps for the teacher. Of equal importance, and perhaps more difficult, is the confrontation that people working with the elderly must make with their own aging and death, and that of their loved ones. I realized the importance of consciously being in touch with these anxiety-producing realities when I spoke about aging to a group of CETA artists who were conducting workshops with older people. Many of the artists said they were unable to function effectively as teachers because of the anxiety and depression they were experiencing as a result of their work with the elderly, many of whom were frail, institutionalized, and cognitively impaired. (Incidentally, these feelings are not uncommon when working with the healthy elderly in the community.) In listening to the CETA artists, it was apparent to me that they would find it difficult to be effective or to enjoy the teaching experience until they consciously acknowledged and, on some level, dealt with the realities of personal aging and death. By consciously dealing with painful feelings, teachers will find it easier to experience the older person's creative process in a more open and full way. With less energy spent on defending against anxiety and depression, teachers will have more energy for relating to older people and for stimulating their creativity. For both teachers and students, the workshop will be more rewarding and pleasurable.

Teachers must also be aware that the elderly themselves have largely negative attitudes toward aging and old people. The 1975 Harris Poll discovered that the young had slightly more positive attitudes toward aging than the elderly. Those older people who do not conform to the negative stereotypes of aging consider themselves exceptions; they do not generalize their positive attributes to their peers. Many older people are quick to make negative judgments about themselves and other elderly; "mistakes" seem to confirm their expectations. Teachers who realize that the elderly view themselves and aging negatively will better understand why older students often do not take risks, why they fear doing something that might result in embarrassment or ridicule from their peers.

Paradoxically, teachers find themselves in a position where they have to demythologize older people's stereotypical thinking about the elderly and the aging process. By breaking down the stereotypes, teachers can help the elderly to take chances, to stretch creatively, and to interact more harmoniously with peers in the workshop.

Understanding and dealing with personal and societal attitudes about aging seem to me to be the necessary baseline from which to proceed into the experience of the arts workshop.

2. SENSORY LOSSES AND PSYCHOMOTOR FUNCTIONING

It is difficult to know whether the negative attitudes toward the elderly come from a lack of knowledge, or whether negative attitudes about aging produce a lack of knowledge. In any case, there is no doubt that there exist many myths and stereotypes about aging and the old. In order to have realistic expectations and to work effectively with the elderly, the artist must have basic information about the aging process.

When we are dealing with the arts, we are dealing with the senses. The teacher must be aware that as people age they suffer increasing sensory deficits. For example, aging brings visual losses. Most people become farsighted as they grow old; their field of vision shrinks, and they adapt more slowly to changes in lighting. Other age-related changes are decreases in color sensitivity and losses in visual sharpness, peripheral vision, and depth perception.

Hearing losses are quite common in the later years. In general, the elderly have less auditory sensitivity, especially for high frequencies. Further, when there is a lot of background noise, older people have difficult in clearly hearing the person speaking to them. Some older people have nerve disorders, resulting in a condition in which certain words of a sentence fade out. Often, they will reply only to the part they have heard, causing the listener to suspect they are becoming senile. For many, hearing aids are not effective. Hearing loss can be more of a problem than visual loss because it makes the old person uncomfortable in social situations, from which they then withdraw. For some, it is too frustrating and too embarrassing to keep saying, "What did you say?"

In addition to vision and hearing, taste, smell, and touch are thought to decrease in sensitivity as one ages. Also, there are changes in the way we sense our body, particularly its position and its motion. Balance is affected and vestibular sense (i.e., inner ear) change makes dizziness more common in old age.

Sensory change is a reality of aging. However, these changes occur and are experienced gradually, so most old people are able to make the necessary adjustments. For example, I recently gave a lecture to a group of older people at a senior center. After the lecture, an eighty-nine-year-old woman who had been sitting very close to me and seemed to be straining to hear told me that she was able to hear only a part of what I said, but that she enjoyed the part she heard.

Along with sensory loss, as people age they experience a decrease in psychomotor functioning. For example, older people have less muscular strength and physical stamina. They also take longer to react to many forms of stimuli and to respond in motion. Again, such changes are usually perceived as occurring gradually and most old people can adjust.

By being aware of the common sensory and psychomotor changes of aging, teachers will have appropriate expectations of the older student and will be able to deal with some of the psychological and interpersonal problems associated with these changes. In addition, being aware of aging-related deficits will alert teachers to the possibility of offsetting them through environmental manipulation. Some ways for teachers to compensate for deficits are: using microphones, seating people so they can see and hear one another, making sure that the workroom is not in a noisy and distracting area, keeping out street noises, making sure that the lighting in the room is adequate, and seeing that people are not bothered by the glare of light or sunlight. In many cases, teachers will have to find more complicated solutions than the ones just described. In each workshop situation, different problems arise, growing out of the losses and changes that come with aging, and teachers have to be creative in their solutions. Often environmental manipulation will be the easiest and most practical solution; sometimes it will be the only one.

3. COGNITIVE FUNCTIONING

Learning: "You can't teach an old dog new tricks." This is part of our folk "wisdom." I've often wondered whether this statement is true about old dogs; it certainly isn't true of old people.

Old people *can* learn. However, they learn more slowly than young people, and they learn best when they are not given time limits. Because of their slower learning process and their anxiety about learning, older people will find self-pacing a more effective way of learning. Also, older students will have more success in a learning situation that draws on life experience and is more concrete than abstract. Interestingly, some studies on how older people learn show that although they learn more slowly, they learn more deeply. They have different strategies of learning than the young; for example, they are less likely to be distracted by nonessential details and are quicker at getting to the basic concept.

Often older people need to be reminded that both the young and the old experience anxiety and difficulty when learning something new, and that given the time they will master the material being taught. Older students need to be reassured that, indeed, they too can learn "new tricks."

Memory: Learning is dependent on memory, and most older people feel insecure about their ability to remember recent events or recent learning. Everyone knows older people who complain that they remember events from fifty years ago, but forget what they ate for dinner the night before. This complaint illustrates the principle that immediate memory falls off more rapidly than the ability to remember items or events from the distant past. And for most people it is true: there is more decline in short-term than long-term memory.

There are a number of possible reasons to explain the decrement in short-term memory. To begin with, changes in the central nervous system prevent older people from processing and absorbing information as well as they did when they were young, which affects more recent memory. Situational factors may have an affect on memory. For example, older people who are ill, depressed, withdrawn, or socially isolated will not be maximally aware of what is going on in the environment and therefore may process and store less information. Motivation may also explain what happens to memory. Some older people may remember the past in detail because it was a happier time, a time in which they were fully involved in life. For these elderly, it may be more pleasant to dwell on the past and to block out the present time, which they do not find as satisfying. Another important point is that it may be easier for many old people to remember the remote past rather than the recent past because they have been "rehearsing" these memories throughout the years. Thus, the memories that have prevailed over the years tend to remain, while the memories of the recent past are sometimes forgotten for the reasons cited above. In addition to absorption, processing, and storage problems, and the situational and motivational aspects of memory, the elderly have more difficulty in retrieving material from short-term memory. As people grow older, they retrieve material more slowly: memories are not lost, they are just slower in coming.

Teachers who explain the slowdown in short-term memory will help to make students feel less anxious when they experience memory difficulties. Also, they can help an older person who cannot remember something from the recent past by giving cues: "Mrs. Jones is the woman who sat next to you, wearing the blue sweater." Sometimes it helps to tell an older person that if they relax, the memory will surface. It usually does. When all else fails, I confess to having burned four pots in two months because I forgot that I had them on the stove. Since I am neither old nor senile, this bit of sharing usually helps my older students to feel better.

It is important for the elderly to know that memory slowdown is a natural part of aging and in most cases is not a sign of pathology. A teacher may also point out that while memory decline happens to more and more people as they grow older, it does not happen to everyone. There is a great deal of variability among the elderly, and some older people, regardless of age, never show any measurable memory impairment.

Intelligence: Many people equate old age with a decrease in intelligence; they think that old people are stupid. Faltering intelligence is another myth of aging. As a matter of fact, research on aging and intelligence shows that in healthy older adults there is no appreciable decrease in intelligence. For some, crystallized intelligence—that knowledge that we gain from the culture—actually increases; this is the case with verbal comprehension. The older person who continues to read, who interacts with other people socially, and who lives in a stimulating environment will continue to function well on an intellectual level.

4. THE MYTH OF SENILITY

One of the widespread myths about aging is that we all become senile. But senility is not a natural outcome of aging. Nor is it a medical diagnosis. Senility is a catchall term used by laymen and doctors to describe such symptoms as memory loss, confusion, disorientation about time and place, and inability to learn or solve problems. These symptoms can be manifestations of chronic brain syndrome, a term used to denote various forms of diseases causing organic and mental deterioration. Chronic brain syndrome includes such diseases as Alzheimer's and senile dementia. In such diseases brain cells are destroyed and do not regenerate, or the connection between these cells becomes tangled. In any event, the outcome is a progressive decline for which no real treatment or cure is yet known. Another disease that produces "senile" behavior is arteriosclerosis or hardening of the arteries. In this vascular disease, hardened arteries cause a blockage of the blood flow, and oxygen is not carried in sufficient concentration to the brain, resulting in such symptoms as confusion, memory loss, and hallucinations. Thus far, chronic brain syndrome cannot be reversed. However, since only five to six percent of the over-sixty-five population is institutionalized, and this percentage includes institutionalization for a variety of reasons, it becomes obvious that chronic brain syndrome occurs in a small percentage of the elderly.

There are also acute conditions which produce the symptoms of senility, such as malnutrition, depression, metabolic disorders, infections, and reactions to drugs. An acute brain syndrome can be reversed when the cause is diagnosed and treated properly. In such cases, older patients can make a full recovery, with the total disappearance of senile symptoms.

Fear of senility is common among the elderly, who share the general population's misconception that it is a natural part of aging. A teacher who knows the facts can help to allay the anxiety many elderly unnecessarily experience when they notice any changes or slowing down in cognitive functioning.

5. PERSONALITY AND THE ELDERLY

There is no "personality of the elderly." Personality is more continuous than discontinuous, and older people will continue to be more like they've always been than like other older people. While the basic core of personality remains intact in the healthy older person, there are some personality changes common to many older people. Some of these are:

Introversion: Many older people turn inward as they age and become more preoccupied with the self. They become more focused on their bodies, their thoughts, and their emotional states rather than on what is happening externally. To illustrate introversion or "interiority," a friend told me about his mother who was in her late seventies. Previously very active, she told her son that she noticed that she was less interested in activities and socializing. As time went on, she found herself experiencing more pleasure from reading, thinking, reminiscing, and letting her mind wander over space and time. She was more focused on herself, and not at all unhappy with the change. Keeping in mind this personality change which happens to many elderly, teachers can encourage older people to express their increased inner exploration in artistic terms. Possibly, too, the artistic and interpersonal experience of the workshop might motivate the older person to look outward and find new interests and enthusiasm in the external world.

Behavioral rigidity and conservatism: Older people are faced with significant life changes and make adjustments all the time. However, they seem to manifest a trend toward more rigid and conservative behavior. Elderly people have less physical and psychic energy and find new situations can make them uncomfortable. Thus, it becomes easier to hold on to old thoughts and behaviors. In a workshop situation, a teacher can often move people away from habitual and rigid thoughts and behaviors. However, it must be done carefully, in a way that does not point out that old ways are superannuated. Optimally, the old and new can be connected in a way that leads to a new transformation.

Intolerance of ambiguity: To stave off anxiety, many older people will seek to impose a familiar structure on an ambiguous situation. Often it doesn't matter whether or not the structure is appropriate. A case in point occurred at an arts conference I attended last year. A unique and interesting poet was demonstrating how she teaches poetry workshops. An older woman kept interrupting her and asking for rules on how to structure a poetry class. When the poet asked her to participate in the experience and learn from it, she was unable to do so. She made it quite clear to everyone at the conference that she felt the workshop had been a waste of time. Initially a teacher can deal with the older student's anxiety about ambiguity by making sure that the workshop and each task undertaken in it has an observable structure.

Restraint in making judgments and taking risks: It is difficult to face disappointment, uncertainty, or failure at any age. However, risk taking is even more difficult for the older person who is experiencing changes and losses due to aging. Not feeling one's best makes it harder for the older person to be confident about making judgments and decisions. By understanding that for many the self-concept is not strong and that there is less of a feeling of mastery over the environment, the teacher will be able to react to the older student with more sensitivity and will experience less frustration, too.

Lessening of social restraints: While there is more restraint in making judgments and taking risks, many older people seem to have less social restraints than they did in the past. A dignified and gracious woman in her early seventies once confided to me that when she reached seventy, she saw no reason to please everyone else. Much to the surprise and dismay of her friends and family, she became quite outspoken. In a class situation, older people are often hard to teach because they are noisy, rude, tactless, and harshly critical of one another. There are no bromides for this situation. But as the teacher becomes more familiar with the individuals and with the dynamics of the group, the lack of social restraint gets easier to deal with. In my experience, acting-out behavior is an individual's expression of a problem such as anxiety, the need for attention, boredom, jealousy, or competition. Eventually, the teacher will understand the root of the problem and with patience and tact can succeed in making the person feel more comfortable.

Interests and values remain fairly constant throughout life: Rarely will an older person with no past or present interest in the arts become a devoted workshop participant. For an older person to become deeply involved in an arts experience, there usually has to be some long-standing or latent interest. For example, although Grandma Moses had never painted until she was seventy-nine and had never studied painting in her life, she had a long history of being interested in the decorative arts, of doing needlepoint and yarn paintings. On occasion, however, a person who has had a suppressed or unconscious yearning to express herself creatively shows up at a workshop; when asked what brought her, she will say "to keep a friend company." A teacher who senses this person's latent interest, desire, and fear, and who responds to it with sensitivity, may be successful in making a "convert."

Gerontological research points out that personality changes in old age might be brought about by a basic change in the organism: the primarily arousal-seeking state of youth and middle age is avoided because of decreased sensory processes and the slower speed of integrating information. Also, the older person finds that energy can be conserved by avoiding arousal. Thus, older people begin to seek simplicity rather than complexity. For this reason, they might tend to avoid new situations, hold on to old patterns, and impose a structure on ambiguous stimuli or situations. Remotivating the older person can be difficult unless the benefits of the new experience quickly become obvious.

The teacher has to "hook" the older person into the workshop experience more quickly than would be necessary with a younger student. Giving structure, attention, reinforcement, appropriate praise, and genuine caring are effective ways of approaching the older student.

Artists who teach creative arts workshops with the elderly are working in a new and uncharted field, where training thus far has been minimal. The problems are great, but so are the rewards of sharing people's lives and experiences. Most rewarding of all is helping people to discover a hidden and creative part of themselves in old age.

A Kind of Odyssey

Lucille Wolfe

I'm an old social worker. Now at age seventy-four, I've spent the past fifty years working in my profession. Just a year ago, in May 1979, I became a participant-observer in an Artist & Elders workshop. Then, in February, my colleague Carolyn Zablotny and I became coleaders of the group. This essay is about how I came to join that group and what I experienced and learned there. It describes a kind of odyssey—my nine years of quasi-retirement, of struggling to remain afloat and find an appropriate place for myself within my profession.

I don't write easily; with a lifetime of hiding myself behind others, it is hard to talk about myself directly, to retrace my steps and reflect on my meanderings. But I feel it's imperative to set my record down for myself and others to learn from. So I'm writing, and at the same time I'm still wrestling with myself to continue because the struggle isn't ended. I will shuttle back and forth between this past year and the previous ones because it's easier to talk of the earlier years even though the struggles of the present have stimulated this effort. It has been a year of crises for me and a year of keener self-awareness.

During the past year, I've been both a volunteer participant-observer in the Guiding Light Group which meets at SPOP (Service Program for Older People) and a part-time intake worker on the paid professional staff of that same agency. Actually the pleasure and support I felt in being in the group sustained me through the threatening experience of a gradually dwindling role in SPOP. The agency, and my job in it, were changing. I was depressed and ambivalent about remaining.

This was not the first time I faced retirement. I had been "mandatorily retired" at sixty-five from the Community Service Society, a large private agency which used to offer individual and family counseling services directly to people in Manhattan, the Bronx, and Queens. In 1971, because of the recession and depleted funding from the private sector, the agency scrapped its entire family case-work division. I was working in the Bronx office and experienced that exodus with the rest of the staff. That made it easier to leave. During the ending phase, we raged and mourned our job loss to-gether, feeding each other little meals of support daily until June. Because I was three months short of retirement age, I was permitted to shift to the Queens office where they planned temporarily to carry a student unit and needed experienced staff to help assemble a pool of potential clients for them. But then in September, retirement was mandatory. I resented it bitterly.

How retire? One does not incorporate a professional self for some forty years only to cast it off suddenly as a worn outer garment. It was my flesh and blood, giving meaning and purpose to my life. Yes, I felt a need to slacken my pace. I wanted longer vacations and shorter hours, but I still wanted my work, and I wanted to be paid for it because I needed the money. So I went job hunting. After almost a year of searching for a social work agency that would ac-cept a person over sixty-five on its staff, I heard of an opportunity to work in a new community outreach program for the "mentally frail elderly" in mid-Manhattan. It was a part-time and temporary posi-tion. And my role in this new setup was rather nebulous. I was hired by St. Luke's Community Psychiatric Division as both their liaison worker and their "loaned worker" to SPOP. Still, I grabbed the op-portunity. It was exciting, too, because my age was considered an asset! I could understand and identify with the stresses older persons were undergoing. It was an adventure for all of us because it was a new agency needing to find itself. Everybody was interested in the job and felt part of a team that was testing various ways of helping the elderly. The job lasted a year. Although my role was foggy and my loyalties were often divided between St. Luke's and SPOP, it was overall a rewarding experience. After that, every year until 1976 I was offered temporary and part-time work at SPOP.

But over the years, SPOP was changing. Initially it offered an outreach program to the "mentally frail elderly." Social workers made home visits and helped the elderly find appropriate housing, medical care, and housekeeping services; they helped them secure their legal entitlements, and they gave lots of warmth and comfort, sensitivity and understanding to their aging clientele along the way. But it was not too different from other agencies. Gradually it was finding its focus, more sharply defining its role in the community as a mental health clinic for the elderly. It hired a psychiatrist as medical director and got itself accepted as a clinic by the New York State Department of Mental Hygiene. With increased professional prestige, the agency began to shift from an outreach program for the "mentally frail elderly" to a consultation service for fee-paying, office-visiting older clients. Social workers with their recently earned M.S.W.'s were asking for a more sophisticated, more intact client group to work with. They wanted to offer insight therapy rather than supportive counseling. Those clients who needed home visits and more protective and directive services were assigned to students and to paraprofessionals. By 1977, when I was promoted to permanent status, there had already been a large turnover of staff. Staff morale was low, and intake had fallen off. Caseworkers spoke of feeling "burnt out" and of wanting clients to "shape up," especially the more oppressively dependent ones and those who required home visits. The kind of enthusiasm I remembered had almost disappeared, and staff was slow in picking up on assignments.

A profound source of pressure was uncertainty about the agency's continued funding. Self-Help, the parent agency, was threatening to withdraw its financial support by June. Generally, clients on fixed incomes were not eager to pay a fee for services. But the state was paying for Medicaid clients, who generally were poorer and less intact. The staff, including myself at times, felt caught between wanting fee-paying clients and needing those on Medicaid. Unfortunately, because of administrative pressure, staff became less interested in meeting our clients' needs than in getting their services paid for. But for our clients, the pervasive need was to be relieved of their depressed and hopeless feeling that they were no longer of use to anyone, even to themselves.

By the spring of 1978, staff was less and less eager to accept assignments, and I, as the intake worker, felt frustrated and hopeless in making assignments. The time was ripe for me to be wondering and questioning if there were not better ways of working with the elderly. It was then that, quite by accident, I discovered a little notice, tucked away in the monthly publication of the U.S.-China Friendship Association, about an opportunity to join a national tour group that would visit China that summer "to study the role of the elderly." It was, I felt, a chance of a lifetime. I went through an exciting, cliff-hanging time to convince the California chapter of the Friends that I was one of the New Yorkers they really wanted. Imagine my joy and surprise at being selected as one of the twenty-four activists who were chosen from among "persons working with the elderly" throughout the country. Our group included gerontologists, lawyers, social workers, housing experts, and a number of Grey Panther workers, including Maggie Kuhn herself, who was our leader. My agency was interested enough to consider adding an extra two weeks to my paid vacation.

China had always interested me. I saw this as an opportunity to witness firsthand a nation attempting to mold a new kind of social human being. I particularly wanted to know how they dealt with lonely, depressed, older people. Well, I found out what should have been clear to me from the start: older people had a continuing role, and an important one, in the life of their country. There were no lonely, depressed elderly people around. We looked in vain for separate hospitals and community nursing homes for the aged. There were none, except for a few homes for the childless aged. We visited one of these, a Miner's Home, appropriately called "Home of Respect" where the retired miners were involved "with pride" in the organization and maintenance of the place, especially the gardens, and in telling visitors about their past. In the country, generally, retired workers really never retired but simply were shifted to other work, often more interesting than the jobs they had previously carried. They were, for example, often elected to positions as arbiters in their communes and neighborhoods and were called upon to settle disputes between neighbors, between couples, or between parents and children. They were particularly effective in this role because of the respect and sense of fairness attributed to elders. They were called in to share what we would call "living history." They called it educating the young about the "Bitter Past." Both the doctors in training and the so-called "barefoot doctors" turned to elders for the secrets of herbal medicine so that these could be passed on. They were leaders in "sanitation campaigns" and in undertaking difficult agricultural projects because of their enthusiasm and know-how.

The elders we met were not lonely because they did not live alone, but always as part of a group, a family, or a commune, and always as equals. This is even written into their constitution. Even the mentally ill in China are not treated as a group apart from the world they live in. I remembered when we visited a mental hospital in Shanghai, we were entertained by "the inmates" who had their own orchestra and played and sang "Oh My Darling Clementine." The relationship of the doctors to their patients was democratic and friendly.

China was an exciting and moving experience. Returning to SPOP was a letdown, and it was growing more chaotic than before. The administration didn't seem interested in calling a staff meeting to hear about my trip, though it was finally called. Funding by Self-Help had been cut off in June. By September, no one on staff had been paid for weeks. Since we were so dependent on Medicaid payments, paperwork had increased to meet state requirements. But the staff had been sabotaging all work, especially the paperwork. A new board was scurrying to find new monies and to introduce sharper controls. We were being inundated with efficiency studies geared to produce greater "productivity levels" while intake had fallen off, and those who had been waiting on a waiting list were no longer interested. Full of my experience of the active Chinese elderly, I felt even more depressed and negative about the difference here.

The staff was being asked for success stories. I could think of none. Staff members were also short of cases and were pressing to carry their own intake. I felt left out of planning, and my function was often bypassed. I also sensed I was being scapegoated. I resented this younger staff that seemed to be meeting behind closed doors at sessions I wasn't invited to. I resented the bursts of laughter I overheard, which at earlier times I knew had been generated by stories that poked fun at the more disagreeable oldsters. Since I was growing disagreeable, I wondered if they weren't also poking fun at me. And sometimes I felt as they did—"burnt out" and annoyed with my clients. Much of this was my anger and resentment at my diminished role; it was my own form of self-hate for being a member of that unwanted and pitied group which had—as it was said in fun—"no future."

In December Ken Berc, our psychiatrist, resigned. It was he who had asked me to come on staff on a permanent basis, he who had worked closely with me on intake screening. I felt the loss of his presence keenly; although a new psychiatrist came in March, for me it was not the same. He was not Ken, especially since, like the new members of the board, he needed to question whether I was turning down potential clients. Far from it. But in the stress of the times we were being given mixed messages. We were told to take on the severely damaged elderly who needed home visits and not to take them on; to raise and not to raise the issue of a fee at the time of intake.

Of course, I bungled the screening of some of the clients, but I was too threatened to admit it. I felt undermined, resentful, and put upon; I was easily angered; and to others I no doubt seemed quite paranoid in my reactions. It was during this period that the files on closed cases were moved from a central spot into a young caseworker's office. I thought that they should have been placed in my office since I, more than anyone else, had need of them for clearance. But someone else had already been put in charge of them, unbeknownst to me. So when the files were moved, I created a scene of which I am still ashamed. I wanted desperately to resign, but I also desperately wanted to remain. I'm sure that all of the staff was feeling very low, but each reacted differently. No one knew who might leave or be retired next. Although all of us were facing stress, we did not meet together to discuss our common problems. Each one was looking out for himself, and looking for how he or she might benefit from the other's stress.

It was at that time, in the spring, that Marc Kaminsky came to a staff meeting to talk to us about forming some writing or reminiscing groups. Previous groups he had led had come from senior centers. Even though our clients might be less intact, he was hopeful they would be interested.

His coming was like a presage of spring. As he talked of these groups and their poetry, I was moved by his joyous appreciation of the old people he worked with. Their poetry was about their lives, their losses, their hopes and dreams. They reminded me of poems written by persons in a senior group I belonged to, the Washington Heights Institute of Retired Professionals, but there were some marked differences. The poems from Marc's groups had added dimension and value because many were group poems woven together from their members' shared thoughts and dreams, which Marc was helping them to find and fashion together. The poems from the Heights Group were highly individual pieces written outside the group experience, though shared with the group. The poems from Marc's group were also more spontaneous, and thus seemed more natural.

I was struck by the fact that, as in my Heights Group, where we were all peers, this group seemed to have a peer relationship to its leader. The caseworker-client or therapist-patient relationship seemed missing. This was like the way it was in China between doctors and their patients. For Marc, group members were all persons, not "cases"; nor did he carry "professional distance." He spoke easily of his feelings for them.

As Marc was asking staff about possible referrals of some of our clients, I wanted to suggest some of the persons I had seen at intake, but I was told only clients already under care could be considered. It was then I realized that I had a great desire to see for myself how this kind of workshop worked. So I screwed up my courage and asked if I might sit in on one of the sessions. To my delight, Marc agreed. But after the first session, he asked me to commit myself to continuing as a participant-observer and to keep a log of our sessions. I consented.

Here in this group, to my problem-oriented eyes, were five clients. On one level I included myself, but I was likewise on another level carrying that professional distance I have noted in others, mentally maintaining it by diagnosing each of them. There was Marcia, with her beautiful face and angry eyes, too obese and tense, picking at her fingernails, obviously afraid of her own anger, afraid that it could destroy others, particularly men. And there were the men: Bob, tall, handsome, sportily dressed, but seemingly uncaring, spouting poetic clichés as though he gave birth to them; Harry, the kind of person who could be overlooked, even in a small group; and Adrian, a low-keyed man who seemed bright and sensitive, but on guard, to avoid revealing himself. I knew him from intake as someone who felt fated to be victimized, especially by the women he needed.

I was also observing their responses to our leader. All seemed moved, as I was, by Marc's introduction. He suggested we were going on a shared journey and a journey in sharing. At that point he shared something about himself. He said that he had known and loved all four of his grandparents, that he had learned something special from each of them; that he had led a number of groups of older people, and that he had discovered in working with them that he generally learned and received more than he gave. This was the magic. Probably for the first time, most of us in that group were being told we *were still important*, and as older persons we still had something to teach, even to our "teacher." I began right then and there to take a second look at these clients, these elders from whom I could learn. And even in that first session, each one began to share something about himself. First came generalities. Then Bob spoke of his marriage—how alone you can feel with another person if that other isn't "with you!" His insight was warmly accredited, stirring from Adrian a comment about the good feeling you have in finding that others have the same problem as you do. Later, Marcia mentioned that Mother's Day was coming up, and Marc suggested that for next time we write an imaginary letter to our mothers, adding playfully, "whether she's in heaven or hell or somewhere in-between."

This stirred my own great need to reminisce about my mother and in turn about my sons. But I wasn't quite ready to write that letter, certainly not for group consumption. Clearly I was "engaged," more as a participant than as observer, but I still was not clear whether I could reveal myself to myself. I looked forward to the safety of taking minutes of the sessions.

Curiously, no one was ready to write about Mother; but, yes, we had embarked on a "journey" in sharing and in learning. During the second and subsequent meetings, I began to experience and understand the meaning of Marc's comments about learning from older people. In this group of elders, there was much wisdom gleaned from life experiences. All were eager to share with one another in a generous and gentle way. In the second session, Adrian vented his distress and bitterness about a friend's abuse after Adrian had loaned him money to help pay the cost of his wife's funeral. The group was comforting and supportive, especially Bob, who noted the ambivalent nature of friendships. He said that Adrian's friend both liked and disliked him; but under the stress of his grief and the funeral, he had vented the negative side of his feeling. Others pointed to the projection, saying that the friend was really angry at the "angel of death," but felt close enough to Adrian to let him "have it." Comforted, and with a new perception of his friend's behavior, Adrian was able to reach out to him again. On talking about this the next time, he observed how helpful Bob and others had been and said that he wished he could have experienced such "guiding light" earlier in life. It was then that the group was christened the "Guiding Light Group."

It was this "Guiding Light" quality that Marc had "turned on" that led each of us to share ourselves in support of one another. This didn't always happen, of course. The light was often dimmed, and the negative, angry side came through. But wisdom and insight were there in each one. My feeling about the five members went through many changes, as these lights went on and off. More and more it became clear that Adrian, though he may have felt himself to be a victim, also had remarkable sensitivity, a gift for generous accreditation of others, and a fine ability to express himself well. It became clear that Bob, despite his clichés and his slick, often uncaring facade, had much insight and a poet's vision: he had a real gift for transmuting his knowledge of the "sportin' life" and the Mafia and the argot of numbers runners into vivid folk tales. And Marcia and Ruth were veritable storehouses of practical information on how to untie the knots we make of our lives. In fact, there was a potential social worker in both of them. More and more I noted that when these other parts of the self—strong, creative, imaginative, practical, and realistic—came through, there was a burst of light in the group. Each was prepared to see, and I myself was beginning to learn, the strengths of the others. The challenge for each of us was to discover and bring out and sustain these strengths; this process supported and secured the frail egos of the members of the group. By turns, and at moments, each one became a healer. Inevitably my own perceptions changed. These were my peers, learning and attempting, as I was, to live with less fear.

A word here about writing. The central theme for the group was writing, in the sense of self-expression, creative self-expression, of finding one's own voice.

As my image of the group changed, so did my perception of individual members. My image of Harry and Ruth underwent the greatest change. I saw Harry pretty much as Bob and Adrian did—the "good guy" or "Boy Scout" whom others inevitably took advantage of. He lacked aggression and was terribly critical of himself as well as of others. Locked into his own feelings of inadequacy, he dared not even express them. So he was bland, a "daydreamer." Easily victimized, he offered little resistance to the painters who, he lamented, had been making a shambles of his place. He threatened no one, and the ladies in the group all "loved him." Although always clean, he dressed shabbily. Initially he spoke up little in the group; when he did, he seemed to have a potato in his mouth.

Every conceivable technique was used to reach him. I felt critical of his being "the Boy Scout," but Marc supported this decent helpfulness in him. Role playing was introduced. Bob became Harry standing up strong against the painters, the landlord, the abusive square dance leader. When Harry was robbed and blamed himself for it, Ruth and Marcia offered all manner of realistic suggestions for future self-protection. I played the role of his "good angel" against his bad one—his savage superego. Harry was urged to criticize all of us, and everyone accepted his criticism. Then, very tentatively, he began to speak up for himself. We learned of his love for the music of Gilbert and Sullivan, and when we urged him to sing, we discovered he could sing with warmth and cadence. Finding that Harry had "a singing voice" was the starting point of a shift in my perception of him as well as others. When we first discovered this and urged him to sing, Bob, who also has a good voice, took over; but this has gradually changed. More recently, in a quiet way, Harry has stopped Bob from taking over. He has also come into his own as a square dance enthusiast. He has become desirable as a needed partner, driving with a square dance teacher to groups all over the state. And he has taken on the role of a "good angel" among us, particularly in relation to Ruth, possibly the most damaged person in our group.

I want particularly to write about Ruth. She entered the group in the third session, and it was from her that I learned the most. Ruth's voice had a perpetual whining wail to it; her English seemed poor; her thoughts were fragmented and trailed off. I had heard talk about her in the past. She was one of those unfortunates the staff usually fled from and described as a "pain in the neck." She told us she had been offered a group as a "last chance." We knew she was a widow who had served as a medic during World War II. She could not be drawn out about her past, though she hinted that members of her family died in the Holocaust. She was full of forebodings about the future. Her references, when she did talk, were always oblique. One never could quite understand where her stories were going because, as if following a road full of unexpected twists and bogs and stopping places, she became hopelessly enmeshed in richly confusing details. She defended herself by leading us away from the real story, the one she prevented herself from telling, and by telling stories about other people, important people whom she had known and who had been good to her. This was her way of affirming her worth. A childless widow with a bad heart and other handicaps, terribly fearful of sudden death, she drew our compassion but resented it. She was most fearful of becoming helpless. But she could be strong and warm in offering realistic and helpful suggestions to others in the group. On one occasion, Ruth confided that she did not like her name, and she had several others, such as René and Bubbles. Adrian suggested that in her writing she might present herself under the name she liked most. The following week she brought in a beautifully written piece about herself as a greenhorn that sent all of us into gales of laughter. Even her voice suited this role of the sad clown, which we learned later had been the only "successful" defense she had ever known for her heartaches. At times she blossoms in her old role as "the entertainer." We have yet to find if there can be a better one for her. Ruth has said that the group is more important to her than seeing her doctor because it gives her a place where she can make others—and herself—laugh.

What I'm attempting to indicate is this: each member of the group has become a guiding light for the others and, if you please, for me. We have grown together. But more than that, I've found myself becoming a peer as well as a social worker. I'm really fond of every member of the group; I had certainly not been originally.

What I wish most—and least—to describe is how the group helped me indirectly through my own ending as a worker at SPOP. I was retrenched last October because the agency was short of funds and could no longer afford a separate, and especially a part-time, intake worker. Though this made sense, I was terribly hurt, experiencing this "rejection" as a measure of my worth. I felt this was not only a matter of economy in a bad time but also a matter of making a scape-goat of an old and experienced staff member who was considered too slow, too unproductive, too "involved" with her clients, and who was disliked by most of the young, newly trained staff. Yet it was not entirely unexpected. Looking back to the spring, I felt that dropping me had been planned long before the coming of a new director in the fall. There had been much talk of not needing a separate intake worker. Flashes of negative attitudes toward me came to mind. I remembered, for example, a talk with our publicity worker. Sometime during the summer, he had mentioned in passing that in putting out a brochure about the agency they had thought of using a photo of me with a client, but vetoed it because they felt it was confusing. I looked too much like a client myself. People wanted to see that our staff was composed of younger persons.

I did not share this view. But later in our group, when Adrian commented on the value to him of having youth—he meant Carolyn and Marc—appreciate him, I felt this was true not only for him, but for me. It also gave me pause to consider that my clients, whom I felt preferred me because I was older, might indeed have preferred a younger person, especially if the younger person was appreciating them.

I picked up "an attitude" on the part of our psychiatrist. Though I found him sensitive, thoughtful, steady, and skillful, I always had the feeling that I made him uneasy. He mostly managed to have short, half-hour conferences with me, although with younger staff he usually observed "the fifty-minute hour." He couldn't under-stand why I needed over an hour, and sometimes two, for intake and screening interviews. His were usually only twenty minutes. He used the phrase, "I've got to go now," with both me and the clients. Comments from clients implied that they felt that he just didn't seem to have the time "to get to know them," though they liked him anyway, as I did. Nowhere did I get the impression from him, as I had from our previous psychiatrist, that he valued my long experience and know-how. But neither did the rest of staff. My participation was not solicited during the preparations for the new dispensation. Quite the contrary. I was left out of planning the new format of records, even of intake; and most denigrating of all, I had no part in planning for the staff seminars in the fall. I will not easily forget the first full staff meeting with students where our psychiatrist gave a talk on the medical and psychological aspects of aging, highlighting some of the problems and the discomfort of youth in working with older persons. Not once did he call on me for my comments or expertise; not once did he make use of my authority as an aging person. It was as if I were not in the room. Was it that he didn't think I had anything to offer? Or was this avoidance because I was leaving?

During that late summer period, I had no Guiding Light Group to sustain and buoy my spirit because we were recessed from mid-August to early October. But we were in session at the time I was told of my retrenchment. In that awful period, I found the group (indirectly) and Carolyn and Marc (directly) helpful to me. I will never forget Marc's immediate feeling connection when I told him of my "retrenchment." He was ready to make himself available to me so that I might talk it over with him.

He also immediately offered me a position on the staff of the Artists and Elders Project on a one-day-a-week basis. He and Carolyn and I would meet after the group meetings for quite a time; they both gave fully to comforting me and drawing out my anger and pain, supporting me and giving me perspective. When I mentioned becoming so forgetful that I let my pots boil over and burn, Marc's comment was, "You sure are burnt up."

I could not speak in the group of my feelings of pain and rejection. I would have felt too humiliated and ashamed and would have considered it "unprofessional." But the group was most therapeutic for me just the same. When Harry spoke of being robbed and of feeling "like a bag of sawdust opened up," I strongly identified and could express my indignation; in the role of the "good angel," I could dramatize that it was not his fault. I could accept writing assignments which Marc gave the group, assignments such as "the hard task ahead" or "when I lay my burden down"—sounds like a

Black spiritual—and write these for myself at home, or share them later with Marc and Carolyn. Doing this writing also gave me insight as to how hard, how painful it is to expose one's pain in a group. The hard task for me was staying "in control" at SPOP through December—carrying new intake, ending with my clients, completing the recording of assignments and closed cases, while running what I experienced as the gauntlet of the staff's rejection of me.

My Washington Heights Group was also a source of comfort to me in this period. Its first post-summer meetings coincided with the beginning of my crisis period, and I was the more conscious of its value for me. This democratic group of elders has as its basic purpose the writing and discussion of papers on various subjects in order to "widen our horizons and to help us continue to grow intellectually and spiritually." No one is passive; every member is expected to research and write at least one paper during the year. Like the Guiding Light Group, the Washington Heights Group has in its own way offered its members, myself included, courage and excitement. When Hilda R., who is over eighty and almost deaf, wrote a story about an antique rocking chair and a sofa talking to each other in an attic, her rueful humor about old age touched all of us. When the almost blind and deaf Bea R. wrote a paper about American and Russian relations, and used a magnifying glass, rote memory, and sheer guts to deliver it—the spirit overcoming the fear—that certainly helped to keep me struggling. In them I see "the view in winter," and it doesn't look too bad.

Well, it's not the end of May, and much has happened since last December. Carolyn and I have continued as coleaders of the Guiding Light Group and have added two new members. We will be terminating at SPOP as a place to meet in the middle of July, and we will meet again in the fall with the same group at a local church or library. It's fluid. It will be good to end at SPOP. I'm now on the staff of the Artists and Elders Project. With the decision to end at SPOP and with the kind of emphasis that comes from the atmosphere and attitude of the rest of the project's staff (they are mostly writers), our own emphasis in the group has been changing. There is a marked shift in expectation toward helping members of the group express themselves in writing whenever possible and toward taping and transcribing what cannot be written. Somewhere along the way I've come to believe that this is what they—and I— want and need: to tell our stories, to give some order and affirmation to our lives. Helping each other overcome all that hinders us, helping each other describe how we cope with our aging, and offering each other some of our own solutions—this is what we are all about, this is the therapy we have to offer each other, even if some of us are "clients of a mental health agency." We each have our own unique odyssey to tell, and we each have a need to find our own "singing voice" again—or perhaps for the first time. But I have to remember that this is not China—so it takes repeated acts of faith and perceptive eyes and ears to tune in on our glimmerings and a joining of youth and age to overcome our fears and draw out our tales.

III. APPENDIX

A Bibliography on Reminiscence and Life Review

Harry R. Moody

This bibliography represents an effort at a comprehensive listing of articles, books, and dissertations that are concerned with reminiscence and life review. The bibliography also includes a selection of articles and books that deal with related themes such as oral history, autobiography, and the use of life history methods in gerontology and anthropology. The literature on reminiscence and life review is large and rapidly growing, and the present selection presents no claim to being a definitive search of the literature. It should, however, be useful for readers of the current volume if they wish to pursue further the issues and ideas presented in this book. The bibliography was compiled from the *Humanistic Gerontology Data Base* maintained by the Institute on Humanities, Arts, and Aging of the Brookdale Center on Aging at Hunter College.

BOOKS AND DISSERTATIONS

Ashley, S. *The Impact of Participation in an Oral History Project on Adolescents' Attitudes Toward Old People.* Dissertation, Iowa State University, 1982.

Back, K. (ed.) *Life Course: Integrative Theories and Exemplary Populations.* Boulder, Colorado: Westview Press, 1980.

Banks, A. *First-Person America.* New York: Knopf, 1980.

Berenson, B. *Sunset and Twilight.* New York: Harcourt Brace, 1963.

Bertaux, D. *Biography and Society: The Life History Approach in the Social Sciences.* Beverly Hills, California: SAGE Publications, 1981.

Blasing, M. K. *The Art of Life: Studies in American Autobiographical Literature.* Austin: University of Texas Press, 1977.

Block, J. *Lives Through Time.* Berkeley, California: Bancroft Books, 1971.

Blythe, R. *The View in Winter: Reflections on Old Age.* New York: Penguin, 1979.

Bruss, E. W. *Autobiographical Acts: The Changing Situation of a Literary Genre.* Baltimore: Johns Hopkins Press, 1976.

Buhler, C. *Der Menschliche Lebenslauf als Psychologisches Problem.* Leipzig: S. Hirzel Verlag, 1933.

Buhler, C. and Massarick, F. *The Course of Human Life.* New York: Springer, 1968.

231

Cooley, T. *Educated Lives: The Rise of Modern Autobiography in America*. Columbus: Ohio State University Press, 1976.

David, D. *The Uses of Memory: Social Aspects of Reminiscence in Old Age*. Dissertation, University of California at Berkeley, 1981.

de Beauvoir, S. *All Said and Done*. New York: Putnam, 1974.

Demotts, J. *Reminiscence in Older Persons as a Function of the Cognitive Control Principle*. Dissertation, California School of Professional Psychiatry, San Diego, 1981.

Dollard, J. *Criteria for the Life History*. New Haven: Yale University Press, 1935.

Edel, L. *Literary Biography*. New York: Doubleday, 1959.

Elder, G. H. *Children of the Great Depression: Social Change in Life Experience*. Chicago: University of Chicago Press, 1974.

Erikson, E. *Life History and the Historical Moment*. New York: Norton, 1975.

Ferguson, J. *Reminiscence Counseling to Increase Psychological Well-Being of Elderly Women in Nursing Home Facilities*. Dissertation, University of South Carolina, 1980.

Fry, C. and Keith, J. (eds.) *New Methods for Old Age Research: Anthropological Alternatives*. Association for Anthropology and Gerontology, 1980.

Georgemiller, R. *Group Life Review Therapy with Older Adults*. Dissertation, Fuller Theological Seminary, 1982.

Gorney, J. E. *Experiencing and Aging: Patterns of Reminiscence Among the Elderly*. Dissertation, University of Chicago, 1968.

Gottschalk, L. et al. *Use of Personal Documents in History, Anthropology, and Sociology*. New York: Social Science Research Council, Bulletin No. 53, Kraus Reprint, 1945.

Gunn, J. V. *Autobiography: Toward a Poetics of Experience*. Philadelphia: University of Pennsylvania Press, 1982.

Hale, N. *Present and Retrospective Learning Needs Elicited from the Autobiographies of 10 Woman over Age 60*. Dissertation, Indiana University, 1981.

Haley, A. *Roots*. Garden City, New York: Doubleday, 1976.

Hareven, T. and Langenbach, R. *Amoskeag*. New York: Pantheon Books, 1978.

Jelinek, E. C. (ed.) *Women's Autobiography: Essays in Criticism*. Bloomington; Indiana University Press, 1980.

Jung, C. *Memories, Dreams, Reflections*. New York: Vintage Books, 1961.

Kaminsky, M. *What's Inside You It Shines Out of You*. New York: Horizon Press, 1974.

Langness, L. L. *The Life History in Anthropological Approach to Biography*. Novato, California: Chandler and Sharp, 1981.

Misch, G. *A History of Autobiography in Antiquity*. Westport, Connecticut: Greenwood Press, 1973 (reprint).

Myerhoff, B. *Number our Days*. New York: Simon and Schuster, 1980.

Myerhoff, B. and Simic, A. *Life's Career—Aging: Cultural Variations in Growing Old*. Beverly Hills, California: SAGE Publications, 1977.

Neihardt, J. G. *Black Elk Speaks, Being a Life Story of a Holy Man of the Oglala Sioux*. New York: William Morrow, 1932.

Olney, J. *Metaphors of Self: The Meaning of Autobiography*. Princeton: Princeton University Press, 1972.

Olney, J. *Autobiography: Essays Theoretical and Critical*. Princeton: Princeton University Press, 1980.

Pachter, M. (ed.) *Telling Lives: The Biographer's Art*. Washington, D.C.: New Republic Books, 1979.

Parlade, R. *Reminiscence and Problem Solving Approaches: A Comparison Study with a Geriatric Population*. Dissertation, University of Georgia, 1982.

Pascal, R. *Design and Truth in Autobiography*. London: Routledge, 1960.

Porter, R. J. and Wolf, H. R. *The Voice Within: Reading and Writing Autobiography*. New York: Knopf, 1973.

Progoff, I. *At a Journal Workshop*. New York: Dialogue House, 1977.

Rosengarten, T. *All God's Dangers: The Life of Nate Shaw*. New York: Avon Books, 1975.

Runyon, W. McK. *Life Histories and Psychobiography: Explorations in Theory and Method.* New York: Oxford University Press, 1982.

Salaman, E. *Collection of Moments.* London: Longman's Group, 1970.

Sarton, M. *A Reckoning.* New York: W. W. Norton, 1978.

Scott-Maxwell, F. *The Measure of My Days.* New York: Penguin Books, 1979.

Shea, D. B. *Spiritual Autobiography in Early America.* Princeton: Princeton University Press, 1968.

Sperbeck, D. J. *Age and Personality Effects on Autobiographical Memory in Adulthood.* Dissertation, University of Rochester, 1982.

Tekavec, C. *Self-Actualization, Reminiscence and Life Satisfaction.* Dissertation, California School of Professional Psychology, 1982.

Thompson, P. *The Voice of the Past: Oral History.* New York; Oxford University Press, 1978.

Vansina, J. *Oral Tradition, A Study in Historical Methodology.* Chicago: Aldine, 1965.

Western, L. N. *The Gold Key to Writing Your Life History.* Peninsula, Washington: Peninsula Publishing Co., 1980.

White, R. W. (ed.) *The Study of Lives: Essays on Personality in Honor of Henry A. Murray.* New York: Atherton, 1965.

White, R. W. *Lives in Progress: A Study of the Natural Growth of Personality.* New York: Holt, 1952.

Williams, R. and Wirths, C. *Lives Through the Years: Styles of Life and Successful Aging.* New York: Atherton, 1965.

ARTICLES

Baum, W. "The Therapeutic Value of Oral History," *International Journal of Aging and Human Development* 12(1) (1980-81): 49-53.

Boylin, W., Gordon, S. K., and Nehrke, M. F. "Reminiscing and Ego Integrity in Institutionalized Elderly Males," *Gerontologist* 16(2) (1976): 118-124.

Brown, R. and Kulik, J. "Flashbulb Memories," *Cognition* 5 (1977): 73-99.

Buhler, C. "The Curve of Life as Studied in Biographies," *Journal of Applied Psychology* 19 (1935): 405-409.

Butler, R. "The Life Review: An Unrecognized Bonanza," *International Journal of Aging and Human Development* 12(1) (1980-81): 35-38.

Butler, R. "The Life Review: An Interpretation of Reminiscence in the Aged," *Psychiatry* 26 (1963): 65-76.

Butler, R. "Successful Aging and the Role of the Life Review," *Journal of The American Geriatric Society* 22(12) (1974): 529-535.

Cameron, P. "The Generation Gap: Time Orientation," *Gerontologist* 12(1972): 117-119.

Chubon, S. "A Novel Approach to the Process of Life Review," *Journal of Gerontological Nursing* 6(9) (1980): 543-546.

Cohler, B. "Personal Narrative and Life Course," in P. Baltes and O. Brim, eds. *Life-Span Development and Behavior,* Vol. V., New York: Academic Press, 1983.

Coleman, P. G. "Measuring Reminiscence Characteristics from Conversation as Adaptive Features of Old Age," *International Journal of Aging and Human Development* 5(3) (1974): 281-294.

Costa, P. T. and Kastenbaum, R. "Some Aspects of Memories and Ambitions in Centenarians," *Journal of Genetic Psychology* 110(1) (1967): 3-16.

Crapanzano, V. "The Life History of Anthropological Field Work," *Anthropology and Humanism Quarterly* 2(2-3) (1977): 3-7.

D'Azevedo, W. L. "Uses of the Past in Gola Discourse," *Journal of African History* 3 (1962): 11-34.

Ebersole, P. "Reminiscing," *American Journal of Nursing* 79 (1976): 1304-1305.

Ebersole, P. "Problems of Group Reminiscing with Institutionalized Aged," *Journal of Gerontological Nursing* 2 (1976): 23-27.

Emlet, C. "Reminiscence: A Psychosocial Approach to Institutionalized Aged," *American Health Care Association Journal* 5(5) (1979): 19-22.

Erikson, E. "Reflections on Dr. Borg's Life Cycle," In E. Erikson, ed. *Adulthood.* New York: W. W. Norton, 1978.

Fallot, R. "The Impact on Mood of Verbal Reminiscing in Later Adulthood," *International Journal of Aging and Human Development* 10(4) (1979-80): 385-400.

Finkielkraut, A. "Desire in Autobiography," *Genre* (March/June, 1973): 220-232.

Frenkel-Brunswik, E. "Adjustments and Reorientation in the Course of the Life Span," in B. L. Neugarten, ed. *Middle Age and Aging.* Chicago: University of Chicago Press, 1968.

Giambra, L. M. "Daydreaming about the Past: The Time Setting of Spontaneous Thought Intrusion," *Gerontologist* 17(1) (1977): 35-38.

Gluck, S. "What's So Special About Women? Women's Oral History," *Frontiers* 2(2) (1979): 3-14.

Hala, M. "Reminiscence Group Therapy Project," *Journal of Gerontological Nursing* 1(3) (1975): 35-41.

Harris, R. and Harris, S. "Therapeutic Uses of Oral History Techniques in Medicine," *International Journal of Aging and Human Development* 12(1) (1980-81): 27-34.

Havighurst, R. J. and Glasser, R. "An Exploratory Study of Reminiscence," *Journal of Gerontology* 27(2) (1972): 245-253.

Hendrickson, A. "Geriatric Autobiographical Sketch—Second Installment," *Gerontologist* 14 (August, 1974): 356-357.

Huasman, C. "Life Review Therapy," *Journal of Gerontological Social Work* 3(2) (1980): 31-37.

Hughston, G. and Merriam, S. "Reminiscence: A Nonformal Technique for Improving Cognitive Functioning in the Aged," *International Journal of Aging and Human Development* 15(2) (1982): 139-149.

Ingersoll, B. and Goodman, L. "History Comes Alive: Facilitating Reminiscence in a Group of Institutionalized Elderly," *Journal of Gerontological Social Work* 2(4) (1980): 303-319.

Kaminsky, M. "Pictures from the Past: The Uses of Reminiscence in Casework with the Elderly," *Journal of Gerontological Social Work* 1(1) (1978): 19-31.

Kaufman, S. "Cultural Components of Identity in Old Age: A Case Study," *Ethos* 9(1) (1981): 51-87.

Kiernat, J. "The Use of Life Review Activity with Confused Nursing Home Residents," *American Journal of Occupational Therapy* 33(5) (1979): 306-310.

Labov, W. and Waletzky, J. "Narrative Analysis: Oral Versions of Personal Experience in J. P. Helm, ed. *Essays on Verbal and Visual Arts.* Seattle: University of Washington Press, 1967.

Lesser, J. et al. "Reminiscence Group Therapy with Psychotic In-Patients," *Gerontologist* 21(3) (1981): 291-296.

Lewis, C. N. "Reminiscing and Self-Concept in Old Age," *Journal of Gerontology* 26(2) (1971): 240-243.

Lewis, C. N. "The Adaptive Value of Reminiscing in Old Age," *Journal of Geriatric Psychiatry* 6(1) (1973): 117-121.

Lewis, M. I. and Butler, R. N. "Life Review Therapy: Putting Memories to Work in Individual and Group Psychotherapy," *Geriatrics* 29(11) (1974): 165-173.

Lieberman, M. A. and Falk, J. M. "The Remembered Past as a Source of Data for Research on the Life Cycle," *Human Development* 14 (1971): 132-141.

Linn, M. W. "Perceptions of Childhood: Present Functioning and Past Events," *Journal of Gerontology* 28(2) (1973): 202-206.

Liton, J. and Olstein, S. C. "Therapeutic Aspects of Reminiscence," *Social Casework* 50(1969): 263-268.

LoGergo, M. "Three Ways of Reminiscence in Theory and Practice," *International Journal of Aging and Human Development* 12(1) (1980-81): 39-48.

Mandel, B. J. "The Autobiographer's Art," *Journal of Aesthetics and Art Criticism* 27 (1968): 215-226.

Marias, J. "Generations: The Concept," in D. Sills, ed. *Encyclopedia of the Social Sciences* Vol. VI. New York: Macmillan-Free Press, 1968.

McMahon, A. W. and Rhudick, P. J. "Reminiscing in the Aged: An Adaptational Response," in S. Lewin and R. U. Kahana, eds. *Psychodynamic Studies on Aging: Creativity, Reminiscing and Dying*. New York: International Universities Press, 1967.

McMahon, A. W. and Rhudick, P. J. "Reminiscing: Adaptational Significance in the Aged," *Archives of General Psychiatry* 10(1964): 292-298.

Merriam, S. "The Concept and Function of Reminiscence: A Review of the Research," *Gerontologist* 20(5) (1980): 604-609.

Mintz, S. W. "The Anthropological Interview and the Life History," *Oral History Review* (1979): 18-26.

Myerhoff, B. and Tufte, V. "Life History as Integration: An Essay on an Experiential Model," *Gerontologist* 15 (1975): 541-543.

Myerhoff, B. "Life History Among the Elderly: Performance, Visibility, and Re-Membering," in K. Back, ed. *Life Course: Integrative Theories and Exemplary Populations*. Boulder, Colorado: Westview Press, 1980.

Myerhoff, B. "Telling One's Story," *The Center Magazine* 13(2) (1980): 22-40.

Myerhoff, B. "Re-Membered Lives," *Parabola: Myth and the Quest for Meaning* 5(1) (1980): 22-40.

Neisser, U. "Memory: What are the Important Questions?" in U. Neisser, ed. *Memory Observed: Remembering in Natural Context*. San Francisco: H. Freeman, 1982.

Noyes, R. and Kletti, R. "Panoramic Memory: A Response to Threat of Death," *Omega* 8(3) (1977): 181-194.

Olney, J. "Biography, Autobiography, and the Life Course," In K. Back, ed. *Life Course*.

Otto, S. "Zum Desiderat einer Kritik der historische Vernunft und Zur Theorie der Autobiographie," *Studia Humanitatis* (Munich, 1973): 221-235.

Perrotta, P. and Meacham, J. "Can a Reminiscing Intervention Alter Depression and Self-Esteem?" *International Journal of Aging and Human Development* 14(1) (1981-82): 23-29.

Perun, P. J. and Bielby, D. D. V. "Structure and Dynamics of the Individual Life Course," in K. Back, ed. *Life Course*.

Pincus, A. "Reminiscence in Aging and Its Implications for Social Work Practice," *Social Work* 15(3) (1970): 47-53.

Revere, V. and Tobin, S. "Myth and Reality: The Older Person's Relationship to His Past," *International Journal of Aging and Human Development* 12(1) (1980-81): 15-26.

Romaniuk, M. "Review: Reminiscence and the Second Half of Life," *Experimental Aging Research* 7 (1981): 315-335.

Romaniuk, M. and Romaniuk, J. G. "Looking Back: An Analysis of Reminiscence Functions and Triggers," *Experimental Aging Research* 7 (1981): 477-489.

Romaniuk, M. and Romaniuk, J. G. "Life Events and Reminiscence: A Comparison of Young and Old Adults," *Imagination, Cognition and Personality* 2 (1982-83): 125-136.

Riegel, K. F. "The Recall of Historical Events." *Behavioral Science* 18 (1973): 354-363.

Ryant, C. "Comment: Oral History and Gerontology," *Gerontologist* 21(1) (1981): 104-105.

Ryden, M. "Nursing Intervention in Support of Reminiscence," *Journal of Gerontological Nursing* 7(8) (1981): 461-463.

Sandell, S. "Reminiscence and Movement Therapy with the Aged," *Art Psychotherapy* 5(4) (1978): 217-221.

Shaw, B. "Life History Writing in Anthropology: A Methodological Review," *Mankind* 12(3): 226-233.

Spero, M. H. "Confronting Death and the Concept of Life Review: The Talmudic Approach," *Omega* 12(1) (1981-82): 37-43.

Thorndick, E. L. "Autobiography," in C. D. Murchison, ed. *A History of Psychology in Autobiography* Vol. 3. Worcester, Massachusetts: Clark University Press, 1936.

Tobin, S. and Etigson, E. "Effects of Stress on Earliest Memory," *Archives of General Psychiatry* 19(4) (1968): 435-444.

Watson, L. C. "Understanding a Life History as a Subjective Document: Hermeneutical and Phenomenological Perspectives," *Ethos* 4 (1976): 95-131.

Wrye, H. and Churilla, J. "Looking Inward, Looking Backward: Reminiscence and the Life Review," *Frontiers: A Journal of Women's Studies* 2(2) (1979): 77-84.

IV. NOTES

Notes

Introduction: A Time for Reclaiming the Past

1. Robert Butler, "The Life Review: An Interpretation of Reminiscence in the Aged," *Psychiatry* 26 (1963): 65-76.

I. MODES OF PRACTICE

A Stage for Memory: Living History Plays by Older Adults

1. The workshops at Hodson were funded by the Bronx Council on the Arts, Project SPEAR (Senior Program in Education, Art, and Recreation), and the Artists & Elders Project.

At the Center of the Story

1. John S. Dunne, *Time and Myth; A Meditation on Storytelling as an Exploration of Life and Death* (New York: Doubleday, 1973), pp. 2-3.
2. The Arts and Humanities Resource Center of Cincinnati is partially funded by the Ohio Program in the Humanities.
3. Carl G. Jung, *The Spirit in Man, Art, and Literature* (Princeton, New Jersey: Princeton University Press, 1966), pp. 82-83.

Tapping the Legacy

1. The resultant book, called *Over the Years*, is one of eight Artists & Elders Project books published between 1980 and 1982.

Heal, Body, Heal: Invocations to Hope and Health

1. All the poems quoted in this essay were originally published in *Transitions*, the patient newspaper of the Burke Rehabilitation Center, which is a transitional place for acute care patients who need rehabilitation to gain mobility and independence. The workshops were conducted under grants from Poets & Writers, Inc.

Minerva's Doll

1. This interview, "A Window Was Opened to Me," was published in *Teachers & Writers* 12(1): 12-14.

II. CONCEPTS AND REFLECTIONS

The Uses of Reminiscence

1. Quoted in Robert Butler, "The Life Review: An Interpretation of Reminiscence in the Aged," *Psychiatry* 26 (1963): 65.

2. Helen Lampe, "Diagnostic Considerations in Casework with Aged Clients," *Social Casework* May-June 1961, p. 240.

3. Theodore Lidz, *The Person: His Development Throughout the Life Cycle* (New York and London: Basic Books, 1968), p. 487.

4. Allen Pincus, "Reminiscence in Aging and Its Implications for Social Work Practice," *Social Work* 10 (1970): 47.

5. A. D. Smith, "Aging and Interference with Memory," *Journal of Gerontology* 30 (1975): 319.

6. A. D. Smith, p. 323.

7. Arthur McMahon and Paul Rhudick, "Reminiscing: Adaptational Significance in the Aged," *Archives of General Psychiatry* March 1964, p. 294.

8. P. A. Moenster, "Learning and Memory in Relation to Age," *Journal of Gerontology* 27 (1972): 362.

9. Moenster, pp. 362–363.

10. K. W. Schaie, "Translations in Gerontology—From Lab to Life: Intellectual Functioning," *American Psychologist* 29 (1974): 804.

11. Moenster, p. 361.

12. Ibid.

13. Ibid.

14. Schaie, p. 804.

15. Schaie, p. 802.

16. Ibid.

17. Robert Butler, "Psychiatry and the Elderly," *American Journal of Psychiatry* September 1975, p. 899.

18. C. S. Ford, "Ego Adaptive Mechanisms in Older Persons," *Social Casework* 46 (1965): 16.

19. Muriel Oberleder, "Emotional Breakdowns in Elderly People," *Hospital and Community Psychiatry* July 1969, p. 23.

20. Ibid.

21. Robert Butler and Myrna Lewis, *Aging and Mental Health* (Saint Lewis: C. V. Mosby, 1963), p. 42.

22. M. L. Blank, "Recent Research Findings on Practice with the Aging," *Social Casework* 52 (1972): 385.

23. Ibid.

24. McMahon and Rhudick, "Reminiscing: Adaptational Significance in the Aged," p. 294.

25. Ibid.

26. Ibid.

27. Edward Bibring, "The Mechanism of Depression," in Gaylin, ed., *The Meaning of Despair* (New York: Science House, 1968), p. 163.

28. McMahon and Rhudick, "Reminiscing: Adaptational Significance in the Aged," p. 294.

29. Ibid.

30. Ibid.

31. Butler, "The Life Review: An Interpretation of Reminiscing in the Aged," p. 65.

32. Ibid.

33. Blank, p. 387.

34. Robert Butler, "Discussion," in Levin and Kahana, eds., *Psychodynamic Studies in Aging* (New York: International Universities Press, 1967), p. 199.

35. Butler and Lewis, p. 43.

36. Robert Butler, "The Destiny of Creativity in Later Life," in Levin and Kahana, eds., *Psychodynamic Studies in Aging* (New York: International Universities Press, 1967), p. 28.

37. Erik Erikson, *Childhood and Society* (New York: W. W. Norton, 1963), p. 268.

38. Erikson, p. 269.

39. Butler, "The Destiny of Creativity in Later Life," p. 28.

40. Butler, "The Life Review: An Interpretation of Reminiscing in the Aged," p. 67 ff.

41. Butler, "Psychiatry and the Elderly," p. 899.

42. Arthur McMahon and Paul Rhudick, "Reminiscing in the Aged: An Adaptational Response," in Levin and Kahana, eds., *Psychodynamic Studies in Aging* (New York: International Universities Press, 1967), p. 66.

43. McMahon and Rhudick, "Reminiscing in the Aged: An Adaptational Response," p. 78.

44. Ibid.

45. McMahon and Rhudick, "Reminiscing: Adaptational Significance in the Aged," p. 29.

46. Butler, "The Life Review," p. 70.

47. Erikson, p. 238.

48. Ibid.

49. McMahon and Rhudick, "Reminiscing in the Aged: An Adaptational Response," p. 65.

50. Ibid., p. 68.

51. Ibid., p. 69.

52. Ibid., p. 78.

53. Ibid., p. 66.

54. Ford, p. 18.

55. McMahon and Rhudick, "Reminiscing in the Aged: An Adaptational Response," p. 72.

56. Ibid.

57. Ibid., p. 73.

58. Ibid.

59. Ibid.

60. Butler, "The Life Review," p. 66.

61. Ibid.

62. Butler, "The Life Review," p. 68.

63. Ibid.

64. Ibid.

65. Blank, p. 387-388.

66. McMahon and Rhudick, "Reminiscing in the Aged: An Adaptational Response," p. 73.

67. Butler and Lewis, p. 44.

68. McMahon and Rhudick, "Reminiscing in the Aged: An Adaptational Response," p. 76.

69. Bibring, p. 165.

70. S. Beck, "The Phenomenon of Depression: A Synthesis," *Hunter College School of Social Work Study Manual I*, p. 150.

71. McMahon and Rhudick, "Reminiscing in the Aged: An Adaptational Response," p. 77.

72. Ibid.

73. Sidney Tarachow, "Discussion," in Levin and Kahana, eds., *Psychodynamic Studies in Aging* (New York: International Universities Press, 1967), p. 185.

74. Arthur McMahon, "Discussion," in Levin and Kahana, eds., *Psychodynamic Studies in Aging* (New York: International Universities Press, 1967), pp. 203-205.

75. McMahon, "Discussion," p. 205.

76. McMahon and Rhudick, "Reminiscing in the Aged: An Adaptational Response," p. 73.

77. Ibid., p. 74.

78. Ibid.

79. Ibid., pp. 75-76.

Reminiscence and the Recovery of the Public World

1. Robert Butler, "The Life Review: An Interpretation of Reminiscence in the Aged," *Psychiatry* 26 (1963): 65–76.

2. Christopher Lasch, *The Culture of Narcissism* (New York: W. W. Norton and Co., 1979). p. 211.

3. Ibid., p. 210.

4. Ibid., pp. 210–211.

5. Ron Manheimer, "Remember to Remember," in Kaminsky, ed., *All That Our Eyes Have Witnessed* (New York: Horizon Press, 1982), p. 99.

6. Ibid., p. 98.

7. Hannah Arendt, *The Human Condition* (Chicago: University of Chicago Press, 1958), p. 51.

8. Mutla Konuk Blasing, *The Art of Life: Studies in American Autobiographical Literature* (Austin: University of Texas Press, 1977), p. xix.

9. M. Merleau-Ponty, *Phenomenology of Perception* (London: Routledge and Kegan Paul, 1962), p. 423.

Journey Through the Feminine: The Life Review Poems of William Carlos Williams

1. William Carlos Williams, *Imaginations*, ed. Webster Schott (New York: New Directions, 1970; New Directions Paperbook, 1971), p. 138.

2. Ibid., pp. 83–151.

3. Ibid., p. 38.

4. Ibid., p. 40.

5. C. G. Jung, *The Collected Works of C. G. Jung*, ed. Sir Herbert Read, Michael Fordham, Gerhard Adler, William McGuire, trans. H. G. Baynes, rev. R. F. C. Hull; Bollingen Series XX, vol. 6: *Psychological Types* (Princeton, N.J.: Princeton University Press, 1971; Princeton/Bollingen Paperback, 1976), pp. 330–407.

6. C. G. Jung, *Analytical Psychology, Its Theory and Practice: The Tavistock Lectures*, foreword by E. A. Bennet (New York: Pantheon Books, 1967; Vintage Books, 1970), p. 11.

7. William Carlos Williams, *The Collected Earlier Poems of William Carlos Williams* (New York: New Directions, 1951), p. 33.

8. See Bram Dijkstra, *The Hieroglyphics of a New Speech: Cubism, Stieglitz, and the Early Poetry of William Carlos Williams* (Princeton, N.J.: Princeton University Press, 1969) and Dickran Tashjian, *William Carlos Williams and the American Scene 1920-1940* (New York/Berkeley: Whitney Museum of American Art/University of Calfornia Press, 1978).

9. Louis Simpson, *Three on the Tower: The Lives and Works of Ezra Pound, T. S. Eliot and William Carlos Williams* (New York: William Morrow & Co., 1975), pp. 266–274.

10. William Carlos Williams, *The Farmers' Daughters: The Collected Stories of William Carlos Williams* (New York: New Directions, 1961).

11. William Carlos Williams, *In the American Grain: Essays* (New York: New Directions, 1956).

12. William Carlos Williams, *Paterson* (New York: New Directions, 1963).

13. William Carlos Williams, *I Wanted to Write a Poem: The Autobiography of the Works of a Poet*, reported and ed. Edith Heal (Boston: Beacon Press, 1958; Beacon Paperback, 1967).

14. William Carlos Williams, *Interviews with William Carlos Williams: "Speaking Straight Ahead,"* ed. Linda Welshimer Wagner (New York: New Directions, 1976).

15. Wallace Stevens, ed. Samuel French Morse, *Opus Posthumous* (New York: Alfred A. Knopf, 1957), pp. 257–259.

16. Jung, *Analytical Psychology*, p. 12.

17. William Carlos Williams, *Yes, Mrs. Williams: A Personal Record of My Mother* (New York: McDowell, Obolensky, 1959).

18. Williams, *Collected Earlier*, pp. 171–172.

19. Williams, *I Wanted*, p. 21.

20. Philippe Soupault, *Last Nights of Paris*, trans. William Carlos Williams (New York: The Macaulay Co., 1929).

21. Williams, *Yes*, p. 35.

22. Ibid., p. 28.

23. Don Francisco de Quevedo, *The Dog & the Fever: A Perambulatory Novella* trans. William Carlos Williams and Raquel Hélène Williams (Hamden, Conn.: The Shoe String Press, 1954), p. 22.

24. See Francis Fitzgerald, *America Revised: History Schoolbooks in the Twentieth Century* (Boston: Little, Brown & Co., 1979) for the equally dismissive attitudes displayed in American history textbooks towards Hispanic culture, esp. pp. 93–97.

25. Williams, *I Wanted*, p. 16.

26. Williams, *Yes*, p. 5.

27. Ibid., p. 24.

28. Ibid., p. 26.

29. Ibid., pp. 27–28.

30. Ibid., p. 47.

31. Ibid., p. 73.

32. Ibid., pp. 50–59.

33. Ibid., p. 75.

34. Ibid., pp. 57–58.

35. Ibid., pp. 53–54.

36. Ibid., p. 94.

37. Ibid., p. 130.

38. Ibid., pp. 140–141.

39. Ibid., pp. 141–142.

40. Robert Butler, "The Life Review: An Interpretation of Reminiscence in the Aged," *Psychiatry* 26 (1963): 65–76.

41. Marc Kaminsky, *A Table with People* (New York: Sun, 1982).

42. Marie-Louise von Franz, "The Process of Individuation," in *Man and His Symbols*, ed. C. G. Jung (Garden City, N.Y.: Doubleday & Co., A Windfall Book, 1964; Dell Laurel Edition, 1968), p. 186.

43. Williams, *Yes*, p. 33.

44. von Franz, *Symbols*, pp. 186–187.

45. See Williams, *I Wanted* and Williams, *Interviews.*

46. Reed Whittemore, *William Carlos Williams: Poet from Jersey* (Boston: Houghton Mifflin Co., 1975), pp. 213–214.

47. Williams, *I Wanted*, p. 16.

48. Ibid., p. 33.

49. Ibid., p. 44.

50. Williams, *Yes*, pp. 24–25.

51. William Carlos Williams, "Kora in Hell: Improvisations," in *Imaginations*, ed. Webster Schott (New York: New Directions, 1970; New Directions Paperbook, 1971), p. 1–82.

52. von Franz, *Symbols*, p. 195.

53. Williams, *I Wanted*, p. 27.

54. Ibid., p. 29.

55. Ibid., p. 21.

56. Ibid.

57. Ibid., pp. 48–49.

58. Ibid., p. 63.

59. Ibid., p. 87.

60. Ibid., p. 15.

61. Ibid., p. 14.

62. Williams, "Kora," p. 29.

63. Williams, "Kora," p. 7.

64. Ibid., p. 8.

65. Williams, *I Wanted*, p. 34.

66. William Carlos Williams, "On Measure—Statement for Cid Corman," in *Selected Essays* (New York: New Directions, 1954; New Directions Paperbook, 1969), pp. 337–340.

67. Williams, "Kora," p. 14.

68. Ibid., p. 16.

69. C. G. Jung, *The Collected Works of C. G. Jung*, ed. Sir Herbert Read. Michael Fordham, Gerhard Adler, William McGuire, trans. R. F. C. Hull, Bollingen Series XX, vol. 7: *Two Essays on Analytical Psychology* (Princeton, N.J.: Princeton University Press, 1953; Meridian Books, 1956), p. 213.

70. Williams, "Kora," p. 8.

71. Ibid., p. 13.

72. von Franz, *Symbols*, p. 193.

73. Ibid., p. 161.

74. Harvey Shapiro, *This World* (Middletown, Conn.: Wesleyan University Press, 1971), p. 11.

75. William Carlos Williams, *Pictures from Brueghel and Other Poems: Collected Poems 1950–1962* (New York: New Directions Paperbook, 1962).

76. Ibid., p. 3.

77. Williams, *I Wanted*, p. 27.

78. Williams, *Brueghel*, p. 3.

79. William Carlos Williams, "The Desert Music and Other Poems," in *Pictures from Brueghel and Other Poems* (New York: New Directions Paperbook, 1962), pp. 71–120.

80. Ibid., p. 108.

81. Ibid., p. 118.

82. Ibid., p. 120.

83. Ibid., p. 73.

84. Ibid., pp. 83–86.

85. Ibid., p. 83.

86. Ibid.

87. Ibid., p. 84.

88. Ibid.

89. von Franz *Symbols*, pp. 207–208.

90. Williams, *Brueghel*, pp. 153–182.

91. Ibid., p. 179.

92. ibid., p. 153.

93. Ibid., p. 156.

94. William Carlos Williams, *The Autobiography of William Carlos Williams* (New York: New Directions, 1951; New Directions Paperbook, 1967), pp. 95–96.

95. Williams, *Brueghel*, p. 162.

96. Williams, *Collected Earlier*, p. 444.

97. Williams, *Brueghel*, p. 155.

98. "Asphodel," a lilylike plant with pale bluish flowers that was planted about graves in Greece by the ancients as now, derives from the Greek *asphodelos* and appears in the *Odyssey* (XI.539) coupled with *leimon*, the "asphodel meadow," across which Achilles treads after having news from Odysseus of his son, attendant on Odysseus' ritual summoning of the dead. Other spirits who come to meet him include his mother, Anticleia, and Tiresias, who acts as mediator with the world of the dead. See Georg Autenreith, *A Homeric Dictionary*, trans. Robert P. Keep, rev. Isaac Flagg (Norman, Okla.: University of Oklahoma Press, 1958), p. 51.

99. Williams, *Brueghel*, pp. 177–178.

Poetry, Groups, and Old People

1. Rollo May, *The Courage to Create* (New York: W. W. Norton, 1975), p. 19.
2. Hannah Arendt, *The Human Condition* (New York: Doubleday & Co., 1958), p. 149.
3. Kenneth Koch, *I Never Told Anybody* (New York: Random House, 1977), p. 44.
4. *Ibid.*, p. 44.
5. Marc Kaminsky, *What's Inside of You It Shines Out of You* (New York: Horizon Press, 1974), p. 89.
6. Koch, *op. cit.*, p. 45.
7. Kaminsky, *op. cit.*, p. 89.
8. Abraham T. Heschel, *Who Is Man?* (Stanford, California: Stanford University Press, 1965), p. 35.
9. Kaminsky, *op. cit.*, p. 219.
10. *Ibid.*, p. 215.

Realities of Aging: Starting Points for Imaginative Work with the Elderly

1. The training seminar, and this essay, draw upon the following readings: Alpaugh, P. K., Renner, V. J., and Birren, J. "Age and Creativity: Implications for Education and Teachers." *Educational Gerontology* 1 (1976): 17–40.

Birren, J. *Handbook of the Psychology of Aging.* New York: Van Nostrand, 1978.
Brill, N. "Basic Knowledge for Work with the Aged," *The Gerontologist* 9 (1969): 197–203.
Bromley, D. B. *The Psychology of Human Ageing.* London: Penguin Books, 1974.
Butler, R. *Why Survive? Being Old in America.* New York: Harper and Row, 1975.
de Beauvoir, S. *The Coming of Age.* New York: Putnam, 1972.
Hulicka, J. M. *Empirical Studies in the Psychology and Sociology of Aging.* New York: Thomas Crowell, 1977.
Kleemeier, R. W. *Aging and Leisure.* London: Oxford University Press, 1961.